WHAT IS THE TAKE CHARGE 4-STEP TREATMENT PLAN?

This unique, personalized approach to controlling bipolar disorder combines medication and supplements, lifestyle changes like diet and exercise, and learning how to ask for help. Groundbreaking and comprehensive, this book gives you everything you need to implement a powerful four-pronged attack on the symptoms and cycles of bipolar disorder. You'll find an arsenal of tools to choose from, including:

- Technical facts about bipolar disorder and how it's diagnosed
- Real-life stories of people with bipolar disorder and how they cope
- Sidebars packed with information especially for family and friends
- Written exercises you can do on your own or with loved ones
- A comprehensive overview of medications, their side effects, and how to find the right balance for you
- Questionnaires and charts for keeping track of everything from your finances and work history to your medications and hospital visits
- "Tool boxes" at the end of each chapter that review key points covered in each section
- PLUS: A selection of online resources and suggested reading.

TAKE CHARGE OF BIPOLAR DISORDER

TAKE CHARGE OF BIPOLAR DISORDER

A 4-Step Plan for
You and Your Loved Ones
to Manage the Illness and
Create Lasting Stability

Julie A. Fast *and*
John Preston, PsyD

**WARNER
WELLNESS**

New York   Boston

Copyright © 2006 by Julie A. Fast and John Preston, PsyD.
All rights reserved.

Warner Wellness
Hachette Book Group USA
1271 Avenue of the Americas, New York, NY 10020

Visit our Web site at www.HachetteBookGroupUSA.com.

Warner Wellness is an imprint of Warner Books, Inc.

Printed in the United States of America

First Edition: September 2006
10 9 8 7 6 5 4 3 2 1

Warner Wellness is a trademark of Time Warner Inc. or an affiliated company.
Used under license by Hachette Book Group USA, which is not affiliated with Time Warner Inc.

Library of Congress Cataloging-in-Publication Data

Fast, Julie A.
Take charge of bipolar disorder : a 4-step plan for you and your loved ones to manage the illness and create lasting stability / Julie A. Fast and John Preston.
    p.   cm.
Includes bibliographical references and index.
ISBN-13: 978-0-446-69761-3
ISBN-10: 0-446-69761-3
1. Manic-depressive illness—Popular works.   2. Manic-depressive persons—Rehabilitation—Popular works.   I. Preston, John, 1950–   II. Title.
    RC516.F377   2006
616.89'506—dc22   2006006826

Book design and text composition by Stratford Publishing Services, Inc.

For my family,
Rebecca Alverson,
Ed Fast,
David Grayson Fast,
and
Ellen Schlotfeldt
—Julie A. Fast

For Matt and David
—John Preston

CONTENTS

STEP IV

ASKING FOR HELP

PUTTING IT ALL TOGETHER

USING THE 4-STEP TREATMENT PLAN IN DAILY LIFE

PREFACE

Many different people will read this book:

- People recently diagnosed with bipolar disorder and ready to find a way to manage the illness successfully.
- People living with bipolar disorder for many years who hope to find more tools to manage the illness more effectively.
- Family members who just went through the harrowing experience of checking someone into the hospital.
- Grandparents, parents, siblings, and friends of someone who is really struggling or refuses to get help.
- Health care professionals who want to learn more effective techniques to use with their clients.

Whoever you are, *Take Charge of Bipolar Disorder* has something for you. A comprehensive treatment plan doesn't leave anyone out. Everyone matters, and everyone can help and find help. Bipolar disorder does not only affect the person with the illness. It affects everyone who has a close relationship with the person who has the illness. Because of this, this book discusses the needs of the person with bipolar disorder as well as the needs of family members, friends, and health care professionals.

YOUR CURRENT TREATMENT OPTIONS

Bipolar disorder is a very complex illness. It's also very serious and often life threatening. Thus, the person with the illness must use a variety of techniques to manage it successfully. Although some people can use medications alone to get back to a normal life, for many people this isn't the reality. In fact, many people with bipolar disorder realize that they need more than medications, but they aren't sure of their choices. It's the norm for people to struggle for a year or more until they find the correct treatment plan that combines medications and supplements, lifestyle changes, behavior modifications, and the most effective way to ask for help. The goal of this book is to help you find the right combination of treatments for lasting stability.

WHAT IS THE TAKE CHARGE 4-STEP TREATMENT PLAN?

The 4-Step Treatment Plan can be seen as a pie. One quarter of the pie is medications and supplements. The next quarter includes lifestyle changes. The third quarter covers behavioral changes, while the final piece of the pie teaches people with bipolar disorder how to reach out for support and ask for help from the right people.

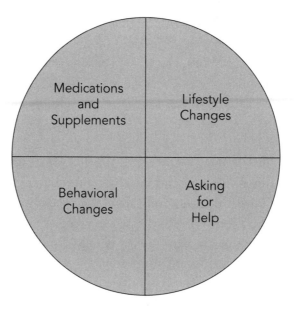

WHY YOUR BRAIN IS DIFFERENT

The first step in starting the 4-Step Plan is reminding yourself that you're treating an illness, not a personal problem. You need help and treatment because your brain is different. Brains are designed to be flexible and responsive to the physical and emotional stresses in the environment. For many people, their brains do this effectively. Unfortunately, the brains of people with bipolar disorder don't function in the same way. To use the diabetes model, just as a person with diabetes can't by willpower alone regulate his or her insulin and blood sugar levels, you as a person with bipolar disorder have a brain that can't regulate itself chemically the way the normal brain can—especially when it comes to regulating emotions. *This is nothing personal or bad.* It certainly causes problems in your life and can be very frustrating, but with the correct treatment plan, you can learn to help your brain respond to life a bit more effectively. You do have options.

The following section is an overview of the book that will explain how the chapters fit into the 4-Step Treatment Plan. Though it may be tempting to skip this section and move ahead, it actually contains vital information that you will need to create your own successful and effective treatment plan. It is crucial to begin by having a glimpse of what is involved in a truly comprehensive approach to managing this illness. So read on.

OVERVIEW OF THE CHAPTERS

Introduction: What Is Bipolar Disorder? This book's introduction explores in great detail exactly what it means to have bipolar disorder, then covers the different symptoms people with the illness often experience. It really is true that bipolar disorder is much more than mania and depression. It's important for your future stability that you know all of your symptoms and how they impact your life as well as the lives of your family members and friends. The more information about bipolar disorder you have, the better you can decide what works for you personally to stay stable. The introduction builds the foundation for the 4-Step Treatment Plan. The remaining chapters then cover the plan in detail.

What Is a Comprehensive Treatment Approach?

A comprehensive treatment approach looks at the whole picture of bipolar disorder and manages the disorder through a variety of treatment ideas from many different disciplines and health care professionals. A comprehensive treatment plan doesn't focus solely on one treatment, such as medication. Instead, it looks at all your needs, from medications, psychotherapy, and physical health to your emotional, financial, and personal needs.

Step I. Medications and Supplements

Chapter 1: Medications and Supplements. How do you feel about your medications? It's normal to have a love–hate relationship with them. Extensive research shows that medications are the first line of defense against bipolar disorder mood swings. Finding the right medications can be very difficult. It can take a long time, and the side effects can range from mild to very severe. This is something all people with bipolar disorder have to deal with. This first step of the 4-Step Plan reminds you why trying to treat this illness without any form of medication can be very difficult. Yes, depending on the severity of the illness, some people can do it, but for the vast majority medications are an absolute necessity—especially for those who experience severe manic episodes.

Many supplements, including vitamins and herbs, have proven helpful in the treatment of bipolar disorder when combined with the correct medications. They also help keep the immune system strong, because the medications are sometimes quite hard on the physical body. There is little evidence that supplements alone can prevent serious bipolar disorder mood swings. Chapter 1 does not discount the people who have achieved stability through alternative means, but addresses the fact that for *most people* supplements are just that—a supplemental treatment that when combined with traditional medications can help improve stability and increase physical health.

Step II. Lifestyle Changes

Step 2 of the treatment plan covers the often significant lifestyle changes that are essential if you want to find and maintain stability. Many people with bipolar disorder learn ineffective and even dangerous ways of managing the illness. From caffeine, alcohol, and marijuana to heavy street drugs and erratic sleep patterns, this form of crisis management is normal and understandable, but these are solutions that always backfire in the long term. As the chapters on the lifestyle changes of the treatment plan explain, many lifestyle choices must be carefully examined and changed in order for you to reach stability.

Chapter 2: Sleep, Diet, Exercise, and Light. The way you manage sleep, diet, exercise, and bright light exposure can have a tremendous effect on the severity of your bipolar disorder symptoms. And the best part of these management suggestions is that they are often free and very easy to implement. This chapter helps you determine what you need to do first, and then helps you to make changes in all these areas in order to create more emotional stability in your life.

Chapter 3: Work and Money. As you probably know, almost everyone with bipolar disorder is challenged when it comes to work and money—sometimes significantly challenged. This is especially so in people suffering from Bipolar Disorder I, which involves severe manic episodes. Chapter 3 helps you assess your current work and money situation (which can be quite scary for many people) and then helps you tailor a plan to create a more stable work and money situation in the future.

Step III. Behavioral Changes

Step 3 of the plan helps you discover the changes you will need to make in order to stop the chaos that is often created by bipolar disorder behavior. The chapters in this section offer a powerful defense against the thoughts, words, and actions that you may feel compelled to use when you are in a bipolar disorder mood swing. The self-destructive thoughts and behaviors associated with bipolar disorder can often ruin quality of life and are especially hard on relationships. The ideas in these chapters take time and perseverance, but once you learn the techniques, life can become considerably more stable and pleasurable.

Chapter 4: Knowing Your Bipolar Disorder Triggers. Bipolar disorder can make you think and do some scary, dysfunctional, and downright weird things. Mood swings can cause poor judgment and impulsive decisions that create chaos and often result in disasters. For many people, this behavior is often triggered by outside events. Chapter 4 helps you discover and become familiar with your personal triggers so that you can significantly reduce your mood swings.

Chapter 5: The Bipolar Conversation. Of all the chapters in this book besides the essential medications chapter, chapter 5 can give you the quickest and most effective relief. The better you learn to recognize and ultimately prevent the often confusing and upsetting things you say when you're sick, the more chance you have of finding stability. The tools in this chapter teach you and the people in your life to recognize what you say and do at the beginning of a mood swing so that you can stop it before it goes too far. This can prevent relationship problems, work problems, and a variety of other issues you may have because of what you say when you're in a mood swing.

Step IV. Asking for Help

People with bipolar disorder often need a significant amount of help and support from the people in their lives. From family and friends to health care professionals, your needs can be tremendous. These needs are often compounded by money problems, lack of insurance, wearing out the people in your life with your neediness, choosing inappropriate people to help you, and ignoring the signs that some people are not capable of helping you the way you want them to. This final step in the 4-Step Plan teaches you how to spread out your needs so that you can ask for help from the appropriate people. It's critical that you have a strong support system around you to help you manage this illness, but it's equally important that you learn to recognize the right people to ask for help and how to do this effectively.

Chapter 6: Choosing a Supportive Health Care Team. People with bipolar disorder often spend more time picking out fruit in the grocery store than they do choosing their health care team. The health care professionals in your life play a vital role in your stability. It's therefore essential that you make sure the people on your team are helpful, compassionate, and qualified to give you the help you need.

Chapter 7: Teaching Family and Friends How to Help You Stay Stable. Have you ever overwhelmed your family or friends when you were in a mood swing? Most people have! There is a fine line between needing help and being too needy. Chapter 7 addresses the skills you will need in order to ask for help from loved ones. It's often the case that family members and friends have no idea what to do when you actually do ask for help. This chapter teaches you how to teach the people in your life what is effective for you personally in treating this illness, opening the lines of communication and helping improve relationships.

Chapter 8: Hospitals. The subject of hospitalization can be a touchy one for people with bipolar disorder as well as the people in their lives. There is often a lot of secrecy and shame when a person goes to the hospital, especially if you did something really embarrassing or dangerous before you were admitted. Chapter 8 helps anyone who has experienced a hospital stay learn to deal with the feelings that result from the experience, especially if you were hospitalized against your will. The chapter also teaches you how to recognize symptoms so that you can stop the mood swing early and prevent another trip to the hospital. For people who have never been hospitalized, this chapter will help you understand what others with bipolar disorder go through.

Chapter 9: Insurance and Paperwork. Asking for help often requires filling out paperwork and making sure you have the funds needed to cover your treatment. Chapter 9 offers you tools on how to best utilize your insurance and understand your options when you don't have insurance coverage. Dealing with paperwork is also addressed—all too often, it feels impossible to deal with the logistics of this illness when you're having mood swings.

Putting It All Together: Using the 4-Step Treatment Plan in Daily Life

Chapter 10: Specific Plans for Specific Problems. Chapter 10 asks you to use all of the tips in the 4-Step Plan to create your own system for treating very specific bipolar disorder symptoms. Once you have done this, you can use your plan to recognize and hopefully prevent bipolar disorder mood swings. Having a plan can make a significant difference in this illness. Stability instead of chaos really is possible if you are prepared for what you will encounter when you have bipolar disorder mood swings.

Chapter 11: Planning for the Future. Did you know that many people with bipolar disorder find stability and get on with their lives? Even if it takes a long time to find the right combination of medications and tools for your 4-Step Plan, you *can* get better. You will have to work on accepting the bipolar disorder diagnosis—it really is normal for you to fight the diagnosis for years, and you may have to change your expectations of what you thought your life should be like. You must let go of the past and accept that bipolar disorder may have ruined many things for you and deeply and often negatively impacted the lives of your family and friends. Once you have done this, however, and have a plan in place to help you find and maintain stability, your illness need no longer negatively affect your life on a daily basis.

And finally . . . *The Toolbox.* At the end of each chapter, you will find a toolbox that tracks the information you've learned. By the end of the book, you will have a large repertoire of tools that you can use, depending on which mood swing or situation you are experiencing because of bipolar disorder. If you turn to the last chapter of the book, you will see that your toolbox is full. There *is* hope for treating this illness; you *can* change the way bipolar disorder affects your life, and as you'll see in the toolbox, the 4-Step Treatment Plan can help.

The appendixes at the end of the book, including resources, a suggested reading list, charts, and a journal, will give you even more tools for the successful management of bipolar disorder.

A NOTE FROM JULIE FAST

Bipolar disorder has a bad reputation. I know this from personal experience because I was diagnosed with the illness in 1995. Many of us with the illness have faced years of pain and discrimination due to the mood swings that make us seem as though we're simply out of control and can't manage to have a normal life. Family members and friends are often frustrated with what they see as our unreasonable behavior, and we're regularly chastised for not working up to our potential, as though we choose to have over-the-top emotions in response to everyday life.

This book is a testament to what I went through the ten years after my diagnosis and how I managed to get my life back despite trying twenty-three drugs without finding relief. In 1999, I had had enough. I realized that my health was up to me. Even though I had been depressed 90 percent of the time and hypomanic the other 10 percent for a large part of my life, I realized I had a choice. Killing myself was not the only option. I could learn my symptoms and do something about the mood swings before they got out of hand. I could keep searching for the right combination of medications and lifestyle changes. I could improve my relationships and live more like a mentally stable person in the real world. Through research I knew what the illness was, but not how to treat it when the medications didn't give me total relief. So I worked on a treatment plan. I knew that I had to come up with something or I *would* kill myself eventually, just to end the constant pain of so many mood swings. This book is that treatment plan.

Today I have a medication that works well with my personal treatment plan. I can write books and am even thinking I'll finally be able to go back to school without getting paranoid and obsessive. Hopefully, I can travel again without getting severely ill. I now have friends who have been in my life for a long time. I no longer alienate them with my out-of-control bipolar disorder behavior. I use my treatment plan every day. My triggers are the same they have always been. Medications take the edge off and help clear my brain from excessive thinking, but I still have to watch my life daily. I still get severely depressed, and hypomania is always waiting for me if I don't take care of myself. But considering the life I led before, I'm now able to function without constantly wondering what is wrong with me and why I have such a terrible life. My family and the friends who managed to stick around when I was severely ill can really see the difference. Writing books on bipolar disorder has given me a career, something I have never had. Before you think I'm different than you are, you should know that I was alternatively depressed, hypomanic, paranoid, obsessive, and anxious off and on while I wrote this book. I just kept it under control.

I had two goals while writing *Take Charge of Bipolar Disorder*. First, I wanted to tell you that you're not alone and that there really is a way to effectively and successfully manage this illness by using the 4-Step Treatment Plan presented in this book. And second, I hoped to help family members, friends, and health care professionals experience—even externally—what it's like to have bipolar disorder, and then offer them proven and easy-to-implement tools they can use to help us stay stable.

Finding stability takes a lot of courage and even more hard work. Having a plan in place that works for you makes the task a lot easier. When family members, friends, and health care professionals are involved in this process, the dream of having a life that manages bipolar disorder instead of one controlled by it can become a reality. I hope you find the 4-Step Treatment Plan offered in this book to be as lifesaving as I have.

A NOTE TO FAMILY MEMBERS AND FRIENDS

While books for family members and friends often focus on what you can do to understand bipolar disorder from your own perspective, the goal of this book is to show you the perspective of people with bipolar disorder. If you're like many of those close to someone struggling with bipolar disorder, it may be very hard for you to truly understand what your loved one is going through. This book hopes to change your view of the illness and help you see that your understanding of the illness is often quite different from what a person with bipolar disorder actually experiences.

By reading about and accepting the many significant challenges people with bipolar disorder face, you may be able to have more compassion when you are confronted with a bipolar crisis or a chronic bipolar disorder problem in your loved one. *Take Charge of Bipolar Disorder* answers the question *What do I need to do to help a person with bipolar disorder find stability?* by offering practical ways to help this person achieve as normal a life as possible. It is especially effective if you can read this book with your loved one and do the exercises together, though doing them yourself is also very effective.

FAMILY AND FRIENDS SIDEBARS

In the following chapters, the main content was written for the person with the illness. You can read this content to get real insight into what your loved one must go through to understand, treat, and finally accept this illness. But you'll also find sidebars written especially for family members and friends. These sidebars will address the questions you may have about the 4-Step Plan as laid out in each chapter, and will help you deal with the sometimes overwhelming emotions that come up when someone you love is diagnosed with bipolar disorder.

You will notice that some chapters do not have a lot of information for family members and friends. Keep reading, however: Other chapters directly relate to how you can help your loved one while making sure you take care of yourself as well.

Family members and friends play an extremely important role in each section of the treatment plan. Management is a large and often unwanted role for family members and friends; the more skills you have in helping someone find stability, the more you can accept the role you may have to play, whether willingly or not. You can do the exercises in the chapters on your own, as noted, or complete them with your loved one. You are not just a bystander in this plan; you truly are an essential part of the system.

A NOTE TO FRIENDS

Friends are rarely spoken to concerning bipolar disorder—and yet you are often the ones who take care of someone with the illness or feel the brunt of his or her mood swings. You're also often more able to walk away from a difficult or impossible situation. If you feel totally used up, worn out, and left out to dry from trying to deal with a friend with bipolar disorder, this book will at least give you the skills you need to maintain a relationship with your friend without losing yourself along the way.

WHAT FAMILY MEMBERS AND FRIENDS NEED TO KNOW

There are a few truths regarding bipolar disorder that may go against your intuition. If you can learn to accept them, however, this can help you contribute to your loved one's treatment plan.

- Bipolar disorder does not cover up psychological and emotional problems; it creates them. When a person with bipolar disorder finds stability, these problems often go away.
- Drug and alcohol use are often used to self-medicate bipolar disorder. The more stability a person can find, the better are his or her chances of breaking the drug and alcohol cycle.
- Friends of people with bipolar disorder are often understandably overwhelmed with the role they are asked to play. If you don't want to play this role, it's your

choice. While commitment to this person is important, your health should not be compromised. Sometimes a friendship with someone who has bipolar disorder that is not well managed is impossible; it's okay for you to set firm limits, seek a counselor or therapist for your own emotional well-being, or cut off ties completely.

■ Bipolar disorder has a high suicide rate—more than 15 percent in some studies, according to the American Psychiatric Association. This is a real threat to your loved one and must be taken very seriously. You will need to know the signs of suicidal thoughts and have a plan ready the minute you believe your loved one may be thinking of suicide. Don't wait until he or she has already tried.

■ It can take a year or more to fully recover when someone with bipolar disorder has a severe episode—especially one that may have required hospitalization. The body and mind are worn out, and the person with bipolar disorder needs a lot of time and support to get better. As you watch a loved one go through this recovery, it is important to have realistic expectations of how long it will take.

■ If you have a young child or a teenager with bipolar disorder, it may be very difficult for you to differentiate between what is normal behavior for a growing child and what is behavior caused by bipolar disorder. As you read this book, you will learn to discriminate between your child's natural personality and the results of the illness.

■ Bipolar disorder is a genetic illness. As a parent, you have done nothing wrong and certainly did not cause your child to get sick. What you do now *does* affect how the illness manifests itself, however. You have the opportunity to play an important role in helping your child manage this illness.

■ Like diabetes, bipolar disorder usually needs to be treated and monitored daily and not just when serious symptoms happen to show up.

■ All people with bipolar disorder act the same all over the world. This tells you that it's not a personal problem. It has nothing to do with how a person is raised or his or her environment. It's simply an illness that affects parts of the brain that regulate emotions.

■ Treating this illness without medications is like treating diabetes without insulin. You would not ask that of a diabetic, so you can't ask it of a person with bipolar disorder. It is not a weakness to take medications: quite the opposite. Taking medications is a sign that your loved one wants to get better and find a more stable life. This is to be commended, not discouraged.

Your Emotional Response to Bipolar Disorder

Bipolar disorder is not an emotional flaw in the person with the illness. Instead, the illness often creates inappropriate and out-of-proportion emotional reactions to events that you could handle with ease. *Your* response to the illness can be quite different. Your emotions are not inappropriate; instead they are acceptable reactions to specific occurrences. People with bipolar disorder can feel guilt and fear, even if there is no reason for these emotions. Your emotions, on the other hand, have a cause and have to be treated quite differently—they are directly related to something that is actually happening in your life. In other words, emotions created by bipolar disorder are not always understandable in that they are a part of an illness. Once the illness is treated, the inappropriate emotions are often more under control. Serving as a support system for someone with bipolar disorder can cause severe stress. Therefore, you may need to seek a psychotherapist or counselor, especially if your main emotions are fear, worry, and extreme frustration.

You Can Use This Book with Your Loved One, but You Have to Be Realistic

It may be that your loved one feels embarrassed or even hopeless at the thought of treating this illness. If you have a good relationship with your loved one, you can truly help by reading the chapters in this book and doing the exercises together. It is *very* important to note that working on the 4-Step Plan outlined in this book can only be done when your loved one is relatively stable. Starting a treatment plan when someone is *manic, severely depressed, psychotic,* or *very recently out of the hospital* is often too stressful for your loved one and very frustrating for you. If your loved one is still quite ill, he or she may simply be unable to show good judgment or to think clearly about following through on comprehensive treatment strategies. This is the time for medications and, if needed, rest. You can read the book and become familiar with the 4-Step Plan so that you can at least work on the tools you can use to help your loved one find stability. Expecting results too quickly is common when you just want to help the person get better. Unfortunately, it often makes the situation worse. As hard as it is, patience is often needed when someone is ill. If your loved one has been sick for a long time and yet demonstrates relative stability and a willingness to commit to a treatment program, then the timing is right to use the book together.

What If Your Loved One Refuses Help or Has a Dual Diagnosis?

Take Charge of Bipolar Disorder offers a treatment plan for people diagnosed with bipolar disorder who are *looking for help managing the illness.* It's well known that up to 50 percent of people with bipolar disorder lack insight into the illness and refuse treatment or have the extra complication of a dual diagnosis (a diagnosis of bipolar disorder as well as a diagnosis of drug or alcohol addiction). These are serious issues and this book does not discount them in any way. Families are destroyed and friendships ruined because of this lack of insight and drug or alcohol abuse. The problem is that those who refuse treatment or are in the throes of an addiction are not in a place to use the *Take Charge of Bipolar Disorder* treatment plan. This does *not* mean you won't be able to find invaluable information in this book you can use for yourself and hopefully with your loved one in the future, but it does mean that you will have to look for help outside a management book such as this one to address the serious issues of treatment refusal and addictions.

When someone absolutely refuses to acknowledge they are sick or refuses to take medications even though their life is obviously a mess, it can be heartbreaking and frustrating to watch, but it's unfortunately a normal part of the illness. In such circumstances, it's necessary to focus on what you can do to get help for the person by getting them into a drug rehab center or committed to a hospital. It's equally important that you take care of yourself if the person will not allow contact. Consult with a health care professional and explore your legal rights in terms of helping your loved one. When your loved one is simply too ill to listen to you or take your advice, you must get help from a qualified health care professional no matter how difficult it can be.

Never Underestimate How Important You Are

As a family member or friend, you have the potential to make an enormous difference in the life of your loved one. As the person with bipolar disorder learns and implements the 4-Step Plan presented in this book, you will also learn behaviors and tips that will encourage and complement the work your loved one does.

Final Tips for Family Members and Friends

- Knowing specifically *how* to help your loved one is more important than showing love and wanting to help.

- It's equally important that you learn what *not* to do or say as what to do or say.
- Your intuition may not be helpful in the long run when it comes to what is needed to treat bipolar disorder.
- Your love is not enough to help a person find stability.
- Caretaking does not help the person with bipolar disorder, and it can leave you tired and often resentful.
- Friends are often expected to be the support system for the person with bipolar disorder, and it's up to you to set boundaries if you need them. You will have to do this in a loving way—people with bipolar disorder are usually oversensitive when they are sick.
- You are ultimately not responsible for an adult with bipolar disorder even if you are the parent.
- You do have a voice. Use it to advocate for your loved one.

Being the family member or friend of someone with bipolar disorder is a tough and often unwanted job. And yet family and friends often stick in there and truly help the person with the illness get better. The sidebars were written so that you no longer have to flounder when someone you love is sick. By the end of the book, you will have the tools you need to help your loved one find stability so that your relationship can be less stressful and more enjoyable.

TAKE CHARGE
OF
BIPOLAR
DISORDER

WHAT IS BIPOLAR DISORDER?

What are your feelings now that you have a bipolar disorder diagnosis? Are you scared? Maybe you're relieved to finally give a name to this collection of complicated and often scary emotions. Whatever you experience, what matters is that you find a way to manage the illness successfully so that you can move forward with your life. This will take time and a lot of planning, but by using the Take Charge 4-Step Treatment Plan as explained throughout the book, a healthy and stable life really is a possibility.

YOU HAVE A DIAGNOSIS—NOW WHAT?

Having a bipolar disorder diagnosis is the first step in learning to manage the illness. The next is getting clear on the changes you're willing to make to find stability. Had you been

■ *For Family and Friends*

Family members and friends can experience a number of conflicting emotions when someone they love is diagnosed with bipolar disorder. You may be shocked. Many behaviors may be explained that previously seemed out of control. There can also be a lot of grief and shame at your own behavior if you have judged someone for erratic behavior. This is normal, because bipolar disorder behavior can be very frustrating. No matter what you feel, remember: Now that there is a diagnosis, things can definitely change for the better and relationships can be improved.

diagnosed with epilepsy, you would need to make quite a few changes in your life in order to stay well. Bipolar disorder is no different. You may have to change your life significantly if you want to find stability and maintain a healthy emotional balance so that you can face the world. Ask yourself this question: *Am I ready and willing to do what it takes to manage bipolar disorder?* Change is possible, and the change starts with you.

Understanding That You're Not Alone

Bipolar disorder may have ruined your life for many years before you were diagnosed. Or maybe you got sick very quickly, went into the hospital, and suddenly had to face the idea that you have a mental illness. Maybe you did some terrible things when you were sick. You may have lost all of your friends, caused yourself unbearable financial problems, lost your job, wrecked a marriage, or tried to kill yourself. You may be despondent at what you feel you have done to ruin your life. Or maybe you have been treating the illness for years but just can't seem to get your life back on track. Maybe the medications have caused significant health problems, such as weight gain. Maybe you feel that bipolar disorder has stolen your dreams, and you will never get them back. Whatever your situation, it's important that you know you're not alone.

All of This Is Normal

All people with untreated bipolar disorder experience significant problems because of their illness. This is just a fact. No matter what terrible and unthinkable things you have done and no matter whom you have hurt or what you have believed about yourself, every other person with the illness has gone through many of the same problems. The good news is that this can end. With the right treatment program, as explained in this book, you *can* repair what seems impossible to fix. You really can.

You Do Have a Voice

The first step toward getting well is to stop blaming yourself for having an illness. Few people say they are a mess and a failure because they have epilepsy, and you don't have to feel that way about yourself just because you have bipolar disorder. Instead, it's time for you to see that you have a voice in your own health care. You do have choices. You do have a say in how you want to treat this illness. The purpose of this book is to give you resources for managing this new way of treating bipolar disorder, to help you talk with health care professionals, help you manage your medications successfully, and, ultimately, help you make the changes you need in order to manage the illness effectively. This isn't a time for self-criticism or shame, but a time for you to feel compassion for yourself for facing and taking charge of your own health care.

TREATING BIPOLAR DISORDER FIRST

Treat bipolar disorder first is a phrase you will hear throughout this book. It means that in order to have a happy, healthy, and stable life, people with bipolar disorder must learn to manage the illness on a daily basis. For people with the illness, management has to come first—before work, relationships, creativity, and life in general. Even though it seems chaotic and psychological, bipolar disorder is actually a very predictable and often very treatable physical illness. Once you start to use the tools offered in this book and treat bipolar disorder first, the illness can be managed successfully and relationships with friends and family can be greatly improved.

MANAGEMENT VERSUS CRISIS CONTROL

How would you define the difference between *management* and *crisis control*? For many people with bipolar disorder, this can be a tricky question, because crisis control feels normal. For most, a mood swing "happens" and then has to be treated aggressively. You then stabilize a bit and go back to your old life and, boom, another mood swing hits you and once again you go into crisis-control mode. This is not an effective way to manage bipolar disorder. It's much more helpful to manage the illness daily with a set and easy-to-follow plan. Nonsuccessfully treated bipolar disorder ruins thousands of lives simply because those with the illness didn't have a plan ready once they got home from the doctor's office. This leads to the crisis-control mode that keeps people in a pattern of reacting to mood swings instead of preventing them. This crisis-control mode can definitely affect a family when a person has untreated bipolar disorder.

KNOWING WHAT BIPOLAR DISORDER IS

Why do you need to understand the technical aspects of bipolar disorder? Wouldn't it be easier to just take the medications and get on with your life? Unfortunately, treating bipolar disorder is not that simple. The more you know about the illness, the better chance you have of finding stability. Knowing bipolar disorder intimately helps you get used to its presence in your life and helps you to see that it's simply an illness that has been documented for thousands of years and that you're not alone in your struggles. The more you know about the illness, how it affects the brain, and its typical and predictable symptoms, the less confused you will be when you get sick.

THE OFFICIAL DIAGNOSIS

The diagnostic information in this chapter comes largely from the *Diagnostic and Statistical Manual of Mental Disorders, Volume IV* (also known as the DSM-IV). This is the diagnostic manual used by doctors to officially diagnose bipolar disorder. If you have never looked over this manual, it's worth your time to go to a library or bookstore and read the section on bipolar disorder.

WHAT IS BIPOLAR DISORDER?

Bipolar disorder is a mood disorder. Mood disorders include bipolar disorder and depression. Although symptoms can overlap with those of other mental illnesses, mood disorders are different, for example, from schizophrenia, which is a psychotic disorder, and borderline personality disorder, which is a personality disorder. If you want to give people

■ *For Family and Friends*

Family members and friends need to know the official diagnosis as well. This is very important if you need to advocate for your loved one, especially when he or she tries new medications.

an explanation of bipolar disorder, you can tell them it's a mood disorder that affects the chemicals in your brain and causes changes in moods that are often not normal responses to outside events. More technically, bipolar disorder is a genetically transmitted medical illness that affects brain chemistry. It results in abnormal regulation of nerve cells that are responsible for emotional regulation. This abnormality in brain chemistry leads to difficulties in controlling strong emotions and periodically causes intense episodes of either mania or depression as well as a wide variety of other symptoms (all of which are explained later in this chapter).

An Ancient Illness

Bipolar disorder is an illness that has been recognized since antiquity. More than two thousand years ago, Hippocrates (circa 460–377 BCE) described the symptoms of both depression and mania, and even speculated that the mood swings were associated with changes in certain bodily fluids. Until 1980, the disorder was referred to as manic-depressive illness. This term captured the two main features of the disorder, but as explained later in the chapter, it did not address the wide range of symptoms that occur along with depression and mania. Today bipolar disorder is seen more as a continuum between mania and depression with myriad symptoms in between.

Some Technical Facts

Bipolar disorder is typically an episodic disorder: Rather than being continuous, there are ebbs and flows as people experience a variety of discrete mood swings. It's also a lifelong illness that is often progressive, leading to increasing severity unless it's treated aggressively. Currently there is no cure for bipolar disorder; with the right comprehensive treatment plan, however, it can be managed successfully.

Bipolar disorders are now believed to affect approximately 5 to 6 percent of the US population.[1] This is a much higher estimate than originally thought. As you can see, you're in the company of millions of people with similar symptoms and treatment concerns. The average age of onset is twenty-one,[2] although it can, in some instances, begin in childhood. First episodes of bipolar disorder after the age of fifty are very rare. It's important that you pinpoint when your symptoms started, as this may affect your treatment plan. Your family members and friends often have more insight into the early symptoms of bipolar disorder and can be a great help in charting the origins of bipolar disorder symptoms.

The Main Features of Bipolar Disorder

The central features of bipolar disorder involve noticeable difficulties in controlling emotions and the periodic eruption of intense mood episodes. It's very important to understand that although bipolar disorder mood swings are certainly affected by stressful life events, it's fundamentally a biological/medical illness involving an impaired ability to stabilize certain aspects of brain chemistry. Bipolar disorder affects people from all walks of life and is unrelated to intelligence, education, social status, ethnicity, gender, or strength of character. Thus it is possible for highly gifted, talented, bright, and emotionally mature people to be afflicted.

WHY BIPOLAR DISORDER MAKES YOU FEEL LIKE A LEAF IN THE WIND

It helps if you think of bipolar disorder as something that affects the mood center of your brain. Do you remember what it feels like to be in love—when everything looks, smells, tastes, and feels wonderful? Bipolar disorder can give you this feeling without the love. This emotional state is called manic euphoria. Likewise, do you remember what it feels like when someone you love tells you that he or she doesn't feel the same, and you're crushed and despondent and don't know how you will survive? Bipolar disorder can give you this feeling of suicidal depression without the actual event. The illness often makes you feel like a leaf blown in the wind by some unseen force. But the truth is that this is a normal part of the illness and one of the reasons it's so difficult to treat. The emotions you experience, even though they're often based on inaccurate conclusions and can be inappropriate or exaggerated responses to a situation, can feel very real. When you make decisions based on these emotions, significant problems are often the result. Once you learn to differentiate between your real emotions and these bipolar disorder emotions, you can make amazing progress.

BIPOLAR DISORDER SYMPTOMS ARE OFTEN TRIGGERED BY OUTSIDE EVENTS

Bipolar disorder is a genetically transmitted medical illness that can sometimes emerge spontaneously—that is, in the absence of major life stresses. However, it's important to know that certain physical, interpersonal, and emotional stressors commonly ignite bipolar disorder episodes. There is no direct way to alter the underlying genetic vulnerability to bipolar disorder. Still, a key ingredient to successful management is to become a trigger expert. Knowing how to anticipate or identify bipolar disorder triggers will give you a decisive upper hand in controlling symptoms. Recognizing and preventing these triggers will be covered throughout the book and in great detail in chapter 4.

BIPOLAR DISORDER IS NOT AN EMOTIONAL OR PSYCHOLOGICAL FLAW

A common experience for people with bipolar disorder and for their friends, co-workers, and family is to misunderstand the cause of the illness and to assume that it's an emotional or psychological problem that can be overcome by willpower. Effective coping skills can certainly be learned and refined, and can contribute a lot to reducing bipolar symptoms, but we must be clear that at the heart of bipolar disorder is a chemical/metabolic problem affecting brain functioning. Bipolar disorder is a medical illness; people suffering from this disease can't directly alter brain chemistry any more than a person with diabetes can regulate insulin levels through willpower alone. The next time someone asks you why you can't just settle down and get your act together, you might want to offer this analogy.

BIPOLAR SPECTRUM DISORDERS

One reason that it's difficult to understand bipolar disorder is that there are many different bipolar disorder diagnoses falling under the broader category of bipolar spectrum disorders. These disorders share some common features: They tend to run in families and may respond to similar medical treatments. Still, it's important that you know what type of bipolar disorder you have in order to make sure you get the right treatment.

■ *For Family and Friends*

Do you feel you have judged the person with bipolar disorder unfairly? As a friend, have you felt overwhelmed with this person's needs? As a family member, were you frustrated and upset when behavior seemed out of control? It may be hard to read that even though bipolar disorder has psychological symptoms, the person with the illness doesn't necessarily have psychological problems that can be changed with psychotherapy or self-control. Once the illness is treated, he or she can work on personal life choices, but until then, bipolar disorder must be treated first. Refrain from blaming a person with bipolar disorder for typical bipolar disorder behavior. You will have to work together to get the illness under control. Until then, asking questions that imply disapproval—*You had sex with a stranger? Don't you have any respect for yourself?* or *You bought what? Are you out of your mind?* or especially the often-asked *Are you crazy?*—simply exacerbates an already difficult situation.

The following section will help you to understand the bipolar disorder spectrum diagnoses. It helps if you're clear that the bipolar disorder spectrum includes all varieties of bipolar disorder, including Bipolar I and II, as well as the other diagnostic categories.

Bipolar Disorder I

When first described in the medical literature, and for decades thereafter, bipolar disorder was depicted as involving two very different types of mood swings: severe depressions and severe manias (states of high energy, agitation, restlessness, euphoria, racing thoughts, and impulsive behavior). Episodes of depression or mania would typically last from weeks to several months, and then, even without treatment, they would go away. People would return to their customary baseline and feel and act "normal." Months or even years would pass during which there were no pronounced changes in mood, but eventually another episode would emerge. This pattern of discrete, intense mood episodes separated by periods of wellness—a state referred to by mental health professionals as euthymia—is now called Bipolar Disorder I.

Bipolar Disorder II

Bipolar II is a version of bipolar disorder with two predominant mood swings: major depression and hypomania—a persistently elevated, expansive, or irritable mood that lasts, on average, one to four days. (Unlike Bipolar I, there are no full-blown manic episodes with Bipolar II.) A study by Judd and colleagues in 2003 looked at the course of bipolar disorder over a period of thirteen years. During this time, people with Bipolar II spent 15 percent of their days in major depression, 40 percent of days in minor depressions, and only 1.4 percent of days in hypomania. The most common length for hypomanic episodes was one to three days, though some people can experience months of hypomania. Thus, the biggest problem in Bipolar II is depression. And over the life span, Bipolar II patients spend three times as many days in depression than do Bipolar I patients. Rapid cycling (four or more severe episodes during a one-year period) is much more common in Bipolar II than in Bipolar I. Bipolar II often goes on for years before it's recognized as bipolar disorder, because it's often mistaken for recurrent unipolar depression. Due to the chronic nature of Bipolar II compared with Bipolar I, it's also mistaken for oddness, moodiness, and the inability to just snap out of it!

Bipolar III

People with numerous major depressive episodes, often with only brief periods of euthymia (periods of wellness), yet no manic or hypomanic episodes, are now diagnosed with Bipolar III as there is a strong tendency for severe manias to erupt when the person takes prescribed antidepressants, stimulants (such as Ritalin), or steroids, or if there is substance abuse (especially methamphetamine or cocaine). It's felt that people with Bipolar III have a genetic vulnerability to bipolar disorder, but it manifests only in recurring depression. The manic "pole," so to speak, is dormant and may never be unlocked unless certain drugs ignite it.

Cyclothymia

Cyclothymia can be described as a low-grade bipolar disorder. It's characterized by recurring episodes of mild depression and hypomania. Please note that eventually, without treatment, many people with cyclothymia will convert to Bipolar I or II—that is, they'll start experiencing severe depression and manic and/or hypomanic episodes.

Hyperthymia

Hyperthymia describes long-term, continuous (not episodic) hypomanic behavior. This may be seen as a temperamental or personality style characterized by gregariousness, high energy, a decreased need for sleep (say, only needing five hours of sleep a night), enthusiasm, irritability, and rapid speech.

WHAT IS RAPID CYCLING?

Rapid cycling is not a form of bipolar disorder per se, but instead is a complication of the illness characterized by frequent mood changes. If you have four or more severe episodes during a one-year period, then you're considered a rapid cycler. Some people experience ultrarapid cycling (also known as ultradian rapid cycling), which may involve a dozen or more episodes in a one-year period. These episodes can range from a mild shift in mood to a more severe shift, depending on the type of bipolar disorder a person has. About 20 percent of people with a bipolar disorder diagnosis have rapid cycling, and it's more common in Bipolar II. It's important to note that rapid cycling can be attributable to drug use or abuse (including alcohol), the use of prescribed stimulants or antidepressants, and thyroid disease. This is why it is important that your health care professional understands how certain drugs affect bipolar disorder—especially antidepressants unaccompanied by a mood stabilizer.

WHY ARE THERE SO MANY PEOPLE WITH BIPOLAR DISORDER?

One reason that the estimated occurrence rate of bipolar disorders recently jumped from 1 or 2 percent to 5 or 6 percent of the population has to do with new diagnostic criteria, especially for the diagnosis of Bipolar Disorder II. There has also been a greater recognition of bipolar disorders that arise in childhood and early adolescence. Additionally, some types of mania are directly caused by substances, including cocaine, methamphetamines, and steroids. Together all of the aforementioned types of bipolar disorder are now referred to as bipolar spectrum disorders. It's thought that Bipolar II represents about 4 to 5 percent of the population, with Bipolar I representing 1 percent, while all other forms of the illness represent less than 1 percent.

WHAT IS YOUR DIAGNOSIS?

Now that you're more aware of the different types of bipolar disorder, you can get clear on your exact diagnosis. This is important because it determines your treatment plan and often influences the choice of specific medications used to treat your disorder. Have you been diagnosed with Bipolar I or II, or do you better fit into a different diagnosis? Do you have rapid cycling? The following section will help you get a clear picture of your exact diagnosis.

Obtaining a Comprehensive Evaluation

The first step in finding your exact diagnosis is to receive a comprehensive evaluation from a qualified health care professional. This may be a bit difficult if your insurance limits whom you can see or if you have financial difficulties, but it is an essential step toward managing this illness.

If you were diagnosed quickly or by someone who is not trained in using the specific tools used to diagnose bipolar disorder (such as the questions from the *Diagnostic Statistical Manual IV*), then you need to see a professional who can give you a more comprehensive evaluation. Were you diagnosed by a psychiatrist, general doctor, or therapist? Do you feel confident with your diagnosis? Not all mental health professionals are qualified to give this diagnosis, so when making an appointment, be sure to ask if the health care professional has this particular kind of training and experience.

Don't be bashful about this inquiry. Competent providers will be open to telling you about their training and experience. If for some reason they're evasive or defensive, consider it a sign that you'd better look elsewhere. These days, there is increased pressure among HMOs and managed care companies for primary care doctors to treat a wide array of psychiatric disorders. While some primary care doctors do a fine job of treating people who are already stabilized on bipolar disorder medications, many do not have the training or the time to conduct a comprehensive evaluation and initiate treatments. Certainly there are some exceptions, and again, it's completely fine to inquire about your doctor's experience and training if you will be getting treatment from a primary care physician. Some managed care companies that are reluctant to refer you to a psychiatrist for ongoing treatment will pay for an evaluation by a psychiatrist if subsequent treatment is provided by a primary care physician. What matters is that you get an evaluation from someone

Peter's Story

Age 40

Sometimes it seems there's just too much to learn about bipolar disorder. In the beginning I just prayed that I would find a medication that worked and I'd get on with my life without having to learn too much about the illness. It didn't happen that way at all. I had to learn more. I wasn't staying well. I realized that knowing what I was up against made it less scary. I learned that hearing a voice that told me to get out of a store was normal. I finally got an explanation for why when I'm sick I act like I have ADHD. I didn't even know what kind of bipolar disorder I had. It was just too confusing. Now I know a *lot* about bipolar disorder. I educate people. They're usually fascinated. It's such a well-known topic now. I'm glad I took the time to learn what I have.

who is trained in diagnosing bipolar disorder and is up to date on the new bipolar disorder spectrum categories.

What Is a Comprehensive Evaluation?

At the heart of a comprehensive evaluation is the taking of a thorough personal and family history as well as noting any drug use or serious life changes you may have experienced. This is why family members and lifelong friends play an important role in the diagnosis. Because bipolar disorder is genetically transmitted, the physician should always inquire about blood relatives who may also have had the illness. Sometimes the information may be well known to the family members, but often it's not. The following may be clues to a possible bipolar diagnosis in blood relatives:

- Psychiatric hospitalizations.
- Married three or more times.
- A history of numerous business ventures.

- Severe alcohol or drug abuse.
- Mood swings.
- Suicide.

It's also important that your doctor ask you about your medical history in order to rule out illnesses that could cause mood swings. There are no specific laboratory tests useful in the diagnosis of bipolar disorder; however, it's often appropriate to run some lab tests (such as thyroid screening) to rule out these various medical illnesses. Some drugs can also cause symptoms of mania or depression. As you can see, there is a lot involved in getting a correct diagnosis, so it's important that your doctor ask the appropriate questions. Equally important is that family members are aware of what constitutes a correct diagnosis so that they can advocate for a family member who may be too ill to think clearly.

■ *For Family and Friends*

Family members play an important role in helping their loved one get a correct diagnosis. Bipolar disorder is a genetic disease, and it's usually not too difficult to find someone else in the family with some form of bipolar disorder or unipolar depression. Statistics show that a child of a parent with bipolar disorder has a 25 percent chance of having the illness. There are often alcohol problems in the relatives of people with bipolar disorder. When someone in the family is diagnosed with bipolar disorder, this often leads to awareness that other members of the family may have the illness as well. Family members often start to remember the odd uncle, the delicate and anxious aunt, the grandfather who could never settle down and was married five times, the wild cousin, or someone in jail who is very moody and addicted to drugs.

Ed's Story

Age 45

I feel like I'm back in school. I have to learn about mania and psychosis and what pills my father needs and how the illness affects his brain. We lived with him for so many years without knowing it was bipolar disorder. He would get mean and nasty and go off in the car and not tell us where he was going. He gambled a lot and yelled at us. He was never violent, but I was scared he would be one day. I thought he was a rageaholic, an alcoholic, and simply a terrible father when he got in these moods. At other times he was so good to us! It was truly Jekyll and Hyde. How could someone so kind and quiet turn into some kind of monster? He finally checked himself into the hospital when he had a fight with a man on the train plat-form on his way to work. He was diagnosed in just a few days. All of these years. It's so sad. He's very different now. We all understand the rage and his uncontrol-lable desire to hurt other people. I realize now what control he must have had. He no longer stays up all night pacing and talking to himself. How we let it go on for this long . . . well, it amazes me. We're all learning about this illness. Having a name and a list of why he does what he does makes everything easier. He's a lot eas-ier to live with now.

COMPILING A DETAILED PERSONAL HISTORY

A detailed personal history is crucial for determining the first signs or symptoms of the ill-ness and its course—prior episodes, how long they lasted, and so forth. It can be very helpful if a family member or partner is included as a part of the interview to get another perspective, especially regarding a history of subtle symptoms and triggers for any prior episodes. Many people suffering from bipolar disorder may have episodes triggered by specific events, such as sleep deprivation while studying for final exams, travel across sev-eral time zones, relationship separation, or taking on a second job. It's important to use a detailed personal history to try to identify any specific and unique mood swing triggers. For many people, the first bipolar disorder episode is triggered by a large life event such as a first trip abroad, starting school, getting a first job, or getting married. These triggers need to be noted so that you can be aware of their potential to make you ill in the future.

The final part of history taking is a careful examination of recent signs and symptoms. Once the diagnosis is made, treatment recommendations can then be offered. Ultimately, you have a better chance in managing this illness successfully when you know your exact diagnosis and receive a detailed plan for treatment *before* you go home with medications. Once you have an official diagnosis, write it in the chart above. As you begin medications, record them as well.

Use this chart to create a one-page easy-to-access history of your bipolar disorder. You can show this to any new health care professional you work with:

Bipolar Disorder History

First major depressive episode: _____

First manic/hypomanic episode: _____

Date of diagnosis: _____

Official diagnosis: _____

_____

_____

Number of hospital stays: _____

Medications tried/current medications: _____

_____

_____

WHY AN OFFICIAL DIAGNOSIS MAKES A DIFFERENCE

The best treatment outcomes occur when people are fully informed and knowledgeable about their illness. In the United States, the majority of people experiencing bipolar disorder go undiagnosed for five to ten years and are thus either not treated or inappropriately treated.[3] Early recognition and appropriate treatment are important in trying to stop bipolar disorder before it ruins a person's life.

Maybe you already have an exact diagnosis. This is great. If you're not quite sure, you may have been able to readily identify your specific diagnosis based on the information in this chapter, which means you can now take this knowledge to a qualified health care professional to make the diagnosis official. The goal is for you to seek out appropriate treatment. As you will see in the next chapters, diagnoses matter because treatments vary depending on the particular type of illness you are experiencing.

It's normal for those with bipolar disorder to be undiagnosed or misdiagnosed for many years. The good news is that now that you have a clear idea of the different bipolar disorder diagnoses, you are ready to examine the typical symptoms of bipolar disorder, so that you can tailor your own treatment plan to fit.

UNDERSTANDING THAT BIPOLAR DISORDER IS MUCH MORE THAN MANIA AND DEPRESSION

As stated earlier, bipolar disorder is much more than mania and depression, and the more clear you and family members are on your specific symptoms, the better able you will be to treat each symptom individually. It would be simple to describe bipolar disorder if it were only about clearly defined mania and depression, but as anyone with the illness knows, bipolar disorder never travels in a straight line. It's more like a crazy corkscrew that moves all over the place. It's normal to feel that you can't get a handle on what this illness means and why your moods are so hard to follow. This is the nature of the illness. Luckily there *is* a pattern to this corkscrew, and once you learn it, the illness is much easier to treat successfully.

The following section describes the typical and maybe not-as-well-known bipolar disorder symptoms involved in the bipolar disorder diagnosis. You may be amazed to find that what you (and friends and family members) thought were either personality flaws or

■ *For Family and Friends*

Family members and friends often only look for mania and depression. This is a mistake. There are many other symptoms in bipolar disorder—such as paranoia, anger, and anxiety—that you need to be aware of as well. Family members and friends are often the ones who notice the symptoms that don't fall into the traditional depression or mania category. You may be on the receiving end of anger or paranoia and may have thought your loved one was just moody and out of control—neither of you knowing that these symptoms are a normal part of the illness.

separate illnesses (such as ADHD) were actually normal and treatable bipolar disorder symptoms all along.

The first step is for you to become clear on the depression and mania symptoms of bipolar disorder. Depression is present in both Bipolar I and II and tends to act the same for most people with bipolar disorder. The main difference between the Bipolar I and Bipolar II diagnoses is mania. As stated before, people with Bipolar I experience full-blown mania; those with Bipolar II have hypomania. The next section explores the symptoms within depression and mania.

WHAT IS DEPRESSION?

Depression is much more than sadness and unhappiness. It's officially diagnosed by the DSM-IV as depressed mood symptoms lasting most of the day for a period of at least two weeks. Many people with depression have dozens of symptoms they deal with every day. Do you have any of the following symptoms when you're depressed? Put a check mark next to the symptoms you want to look for and manage in the future.

- ☐ Sadness, unhappiness, feelings of despair and hopelessness.
- ☐ Irritability, frustration, low tolerance, anger.
- ☐ Low self-esteem, feeling worthless or inadequate, loss of self-confidence.

- [ ] Negative, pessimistic thinking. A bleak view of yourself, current life circumstances, and the future.
- [ ] Lack of enthusiasm; apathy.
- [ ] Loss of a sense of aliveness and diminished interest in life activities that once were a source of pleasure and interest.
- [ ] Suicidal thoughts.
- [ ] Poor memory and concentration.
- [ ] Sleep disturbances: insomnia, sleeping too much, restless sleep, waking up too early and being unable to get back to sleep.
- [ ] Appetite changes—either increased or decreased.
- [ ] Loss of sex drive.
- [ ] Restlessness or agitation.
- [ ] Lack of energy.
- [ ] Inability to work efficiently.
- [ ] Feeling that there is no purpose in life. Asking yourself, *What's the point?*
- [ ] Constant questioning and examining of life and your own behaviors.
- [ ] Binge eating or starving yourself, and being unable to exercise.
- [ ] Relationship problems/loss of relationships.
- [ ] Feeling terrible all the time, mentally and physically.
- [ ] Nagging unhappiness—the feeling that there's never enough.
- [ ] Negativity and meanness.
- [ ] Hallucinations—hearing voices, for instance, or seeing yourself killed or hurt.
- [ ] Neediness.
- [ ] Anxiety.
- [ ] Being overly emotional; crying easily.
- [ ] Distorted thoughts.
- [ ] Paranoid ideas: *People are talking about me.*
- [ ] Reduced immunity to illness.
- [ ] Being overly concerned with the lives of others.
- [ ] Making negative comparisons of yourself with others.
- [ ] Feeling easily overwhelmed.
- [ ] Difficulty meeting obligations.
- [ ] Oversensitivity.
- [ ] Overanalyzing everything.

☐ Brain racing and looping—one thought keeps going through your mind over and over again.

☐ Inability to make a decision—and when you do, it never feels right.

As you can see, so many of these symptoms can be confused with personality problems. When depressed, you may have been seen as unmotivated, lazy, or unable to deal with the real world. It's extremely important that you know what depression does to your life so that you can learn to treat it as an illness and not as something wrong with your personality. Treatment for depression is covered throughout the book.

WHAT IS MANIA?

There are two types of mania in the bipolar disorder diagnosis according to the DSM-IV.

Full-blown mania describes manic mood symptoms lasting at least one week (or less if hospitalization is required). For some people, these manic episodes can last for months. A manic episode is defined by a distinct period during which there is an abnormally and persistently elevated, expansive, or irritable mood. In the elevated state, the mood is upbeat, euphoric, and happy. In an expansive state, the mood is intense, and emotions are shown with no inhibition. Although many people think that euphoria and expansive moods are the main characteristics of mania, many people in a manic episode experience irritability, anxiety, or an uncomfortable sense of increased energy. Full-blown mania often leads to severe social impairment and occupational dysfunctioning, and usually requires hospitalization.

Hypomania is also described as an abnormal or persistently elevated, expansive, or irritable mood that lasts on average one to four days—though, as with full-blown mania, a hypomanic episode can also last for months. The difference is that although mania and hypomania have an identical list of characteristic symptoms, the disturbance caused by hypomania is not usually severe enough to result in marked impairment in social or occupational functioning or to require hospitalization. For some people, hypomania actually does cause significant impairment, but it's always less severe than a full-blown manic episode.

Manic and hypomanic episodes often begin suddenly, with a rapid escalation of symptoms over a few days. Mania is extremely confusing for the people around the ill person. As a family member, you may know the feeling of suddenly seeing your loved one

---

The Difference Between Mania and Hypomania

Mania is seen in Bipolar I, while hypomania is part of Bipolar II. The difference is that hypomania, which shares the same symptoms as full-blown mania, is not as serious, though it still causes significant problems in the lives of people with bipolar disorder. Both mania and hypomania have progressive symptoms. In other words, mania can feel wonderful at first, but can very quickly turn into something disjointed, scary, and completely debilitating.

---

completely change while you wonder what in the world is going on. The behaviors are usually so out of character that people experiencing mania and those around them have no idea what's happening, and relationships are often ruined. With both mania and hypomania, there is a decreased need for sleep—indeed, this is often the first sign that mania is starting.

Manic Symptoms

Mania is a lot more than feeling happy. Do you have any of the following symptoms when you're manic? Put a check mark next to the symptoms you want to look for and manage in the future.

- [ ] Feeling great no matter what happens.
- [ ] A profound feeling of physical well-being.
- [ ] Increased self-esteem or grandiosity; an unrealistically inflated sense of self-worth (*I'm the smartest person in the world*). Looking in the mirror and thinking how beautiful or handsome you are.
- [ ] Decreased need for sleep. You may, for example, feel fully rested after only four or five hours of sleep at night.
- [ ] Increased involvement in goal-directed activities.
- [ ] Having thoughts such as, *The world is just so beautiful and full of possibilities. I can do anything I want to do!*
- [ ] Talkativeness and rapid speech; others have a difficult time getting a word into the conversation.

- [ ] Racing thoughts.
- [ ] Gregariousness.
- [ ] Starting new projects you're confident will change the world.
- [ ] Highly distractible—unable to focus on one project.
- [ ] Hyperactivity, restlessness, or agitation.
- [ ] Talkativeness with strangers.
- [ ] Excessive spending—say, maxing out credit cards, gambling, or buying more objects than you can actually use.
- [ ] Often exhibiting an inability to distinguish between safe and unsafe behaviors.
- [ ] Increased use of alcohol or stimulant drugs.
- [ ] Psychotic symptoms (more severe psychotic symptoms are only seen in full-blown mania).
- [ ] Increased sexual desire.
- [ ] Lack of concern for how family members and friends feel about your behavior.
- [ ] Poor judgment and engaging in high-risk behaviors: reckless driving, excessive spending sprees, gambling, giving away large sums of money, sexual promiscuity.
- [ ] Loss of all contact with reality.
- [ ] The inability to see you're sick even though it's obvious to others; resisting treatment.
- [ ] With full-blown mania, the person eventually can't function on his or her own and must go to the hospital.

According to the DSM-IV, mania can also be ignited by the use of antidepressants, electroconvulsive shock treatments, light therapy, and drugs such as corticosteroids.

What Is a Mixed Mania?

Mixed mania (also called dysphoric mania or a mixed episode) occurs when the criteria for both a major depressive episode and a major manic (or hypomanic) episode are present every day for at least one week. Mixed mania has typical manic symptoms such as restlessness, agitation, rapid thoughts, and decreased need for sleep, but rather than euphoria, there is extreme pessimism, negativity, irritability, and often thoughts of suicide. Such episodes are chaotic and confusing.

IT'S NOT JUST DEPRESSION AND MANIA: KNOWING THE OTHER COMMON SYMPTOMS OF BIPOLAR DISORDER

Now that you have more information on the typical symptoms found in depression and mania mood swings, you're ready to explore the other major symptoms of the illness. Bipolar disorder can seem very random and chaotic when you start to explore these other symptoms, but once you learn the pattern of your symptoms, you can create a plan that treats the illness comprehensively. The following is a list of symptoms that you may not know are common in bipolar disorder. This information will help you as you start to learn the difference between what is your normal behavior and what is behavior caused by bipolar disorder. As you become more aware of this difference, you can learn to manage bipolar disorder more effectively.

Psychosis

Many people with bipolar disorder experience psychotic symptoms. Psychosis is defined as a loss of contact or break with reality, which shows itself in a number of different ways (listed below). While some of these symptoms are intense, hard to ignore, and easy to diagnose, others may be more subtle. You may have lived for years with such psychotic experiences without recognizing them as common symptoms of bipolar disorder. Psychotic symptoms are marked by confusion, disorganized thinking, and often bizarre behavior. The following includes some of the more common types of psychotic symptoms of bipolar disorder.

Psychotic Paranoid Thoughts

Paranoid thoughts include unrealistic beliefs that others are trying to harm or control you—feeling that you're being spied upon, followed, or plotted against, for instance, or that people are reading your thoughts—or the belief that no one likes you, or that a group of people you would normally consider friends suddenly don't want your company and are lying about you behind your back. Sometimes this may involve unrealistic beliefs about infidelity or the unshakable belief that someone you thought cared about you has suddenly changed and now doesn't want to be near you. It's usually very difficult to talk a person out of such beliefs, which is why you need to know the first signs of your own paranoid thoughts. Otherwise you may make a phone call or send an e-mail to someone who truly cares about you that could hurt or end your relationship. What paranoid thoughts do you have when you're sick? The more you're aware of these thoughts, the easier it will be to remind yourself that they simply mean that you are experiencing psychotic symptoms and need to treat bipolar disorder first. Friends are often the recipients of this paranoid behavior, and it's very difficult to maintain friendships when people have to deal with someone who simply does not believe that they care.

Psychotic Hallucinations

Hallucinations are defined as seeing, hearing, or smelling something that's not really there. With auditory hallucinations, you literally hear a voice saying something out loud, as if it came from a real person, but in fact no one is actually speaking—there is no external stimulus. The voice is not experienced as a mere thought, but rather is "heard" in much the same way as you hear anything else. It may be experienced as coming from outside your mind or from within. Also, it can be a familiar, recognizable voice, or the voice of a stranger, or even your own voice (as if speaking to yourself). This phenomenon is not just inner "self-talk"; it actually is perceived as your own voice or a strange voice speaking out loud, usually saying things that are harsh, negative, and self-critical. Though it can be a bit scary, you're normal if you answer these internal voices out loud.

Another experience has been referred to as thought intrusion. Here, often disturbing and emotionally powerful thoughts appear to enter your mind. The thoughts have an intrusive quality about them, but there is not a sense of ownership. The thoughts seem to come out of nowhere—they aren't experienced as a product of your own mind. At times you may believe that the thought has been inserted into your mind by someone else, perhaps via radio waves or telepathy.

The main difference between the two is that auditory hallucinations are perceived as coming from outside the body as a separate voice and are literally heard, while the thought insertions simply drop into the mind fully formed just as you would have the thought that you're hungry or tired. With auditory hallucinations, you may turn around to see if someone actually spoke to you. With thought insertions, you may wonder why on earth you would have a thought so bizarre and scary. One way to know the difference between the two is by whether the sentence uses *I* or *you*. Auditory hallucinations tend to use the *you* form of a sentence, while thought insertions tend to use the *I* form.

Here are some examples of auditory hallucinations:

- "You should be dead. Take a gun and kill yourself."
- "Things would be better if you just got cancer and died."

- "You should just step off the curb and walk in front of that bus."
- "You're a fake and a failure."
- "No one likes you and people are talking about you at work."
- "Your life is one big fat mistake."
- "You're a genius."
- You hear a voice calling your name and you turn around to see who is calling you.

Here are some examples of intrusive thought:

- "I want to die."
- "I wish I could just get cancer and die."
- "I wish someone would murder me."
- "I'm a fake and a failure."
- "No one likes me. I have no friends."
- "I have no right to be here."
- "I'm a genius."
- "I'm the most beautiful/smartest person in the room."

As you can see, auditory hallucinations and intrusive thoughts can be positive or negative, but they're always unrealistic and often very scary. The more of these voices and thoughts you can identify, the easier it will be for you to remind yourself that they're a normal part of bipolar disorder for many people. It's important to know that these voices and thoughts are not real and are not a sign of low self-esteem or personality problems, but instead are a sign that you're sick and need help treating bipolar disorder—especially in terms of managing the triggers that lead to psychotic thoughts.

Other types of hallucinations may be present when a person is psychotic. For some people, feeling that they smell funny is a typical hallucination. Visual hallucinations can be quite scary as well. Have you ever seen yourself get hit by a car and then realized it was just a vision? Have you seen a leaf that looked like a severed hand or seen animals scurry around the chairs in your home? These are all typical visual hallucinations.

Although appropriate medication treatments are the best solutions for reducing hallucinations, hallucinations are also stress-induced. Thus, practicing the ideas in this book can help minimize and hopefully prevent hallucinations. No matter what type of hallucinations you experience, it's important to discuss them with your doctor: They are a sign that you need help with psychosis.

Psychotic Delusions

Delusions are extremely unrealistic or even bizarre beliefs—for example, a belief that you're dead, or have no internal organs, or are possessed by Satan, or are a special messenger sent to earth by God. No amount of convincing or reassuring by others can alter these beliefs.

■ *For Family and Friends*

Psychosis is scary for many people, especially if a loved one's psychotic episode is severe enough to warrant hospitalization. And yet psychosis for many people with bipolar disorder is a very normal symptom of the illness, as are the other symptoms discussed in this chapter. Yes, psychosis is frightening, but it can be recognized early, treated, and ultimately prevented with the right medications, behavior modifications, and lifestyle changes.

Anxiety

One of the more common symptoms of bipolar disorder, anxiety can be present whether you're depressed or manic and can often exist by itself. Anxiety is the most common coexisting symptom in bipolar disorder, as it occurs in more than 90 percent of people with the illness. There is generalized anxiety, which is present most of the time, or sudden, extremely intense surges of anxiety referred to as panic attacks (which generally last only a few minutes). Anxiety symptoms include nervousness, tension, shortness of breath, a racing heart, tremors, cold hands and feet, light-headedness, crying, and worry (such as by anticipating calamities). These symptoms are a normal part of bipolar disorder, and treatments for anxiety need to be included in your treatment plan. Anxiety is one of the most treatable symptoms of bipolar disorder, especially if you discover and modify its triggers.

Irritation, Anger, Aggression, and Violent Behavior

One of the biggest problems with bipolar disorder is that irritation, anger, aggression, and violent behavior symptoms often go untreated until someone ends up in jail or does something violent that may ruin his or her life. Extreme irritability or aggression (for which, later, many people feel much regret) is a normal part of untreated bipolar disorder for some people. Mild to medium irritation and anger, especially with depression, are very common symptoms even when bipolar disorder is being treated with medications, and must be addressed in your treatment plan. Violent behavior can include fighting, stabbing someone, or something much worse. This behavior must be prevented as the consequences are *very* serious. Family members and friends are often a target of these symptoms; it's important that you learn the skills taught later in this book to make sure you don't take your anger out on the people you love.

Cognitive Problems/ADHD Symptoms

Difficulties concentrating or paying attention, poor memory, and problems staying focused on tasks at school or work are completely normal when bipolar disorder is not being managed effectively. This doesn't necessarily mean that you have ADHD or other learning disabilities. It simply means that you need to manage bipolar disorder effectively so that you can concentrate once again. It's also important that you're aware of your medication side effects, since many medications can cause problems with memory, writing, and other attention issues.

Obsessions and Compulsions

Obsessions and compulsions include recurrent, very unpleasant thoughts (obsessions) such as excessive worries about dirt, germs, and contamination; rituals (compulsions); the need to maintain symmetry and orderliness in your environment; and checking your own behaviors (such as repeatedly checking to make sure doors are locked or the oven is turned off). Obsessions may include recurrent thoughts about religious or spiritual issues, such as excessive thoughts that you have just committed a sin. In milder forms, these obsessions may include constantly thinking about other people, checking e-mail or your phone compulsively, or having obsessive thoughts about yourself that you can't control. These obsessive thoughts can be triggered by relationship problems as well as many other stressful life events. It is often helpful to remove the trigger of your obsessions, such as by getting rid of your cell phone or disconnecting the Internet at home.

Overstimulated Symptoms

Feeling overstimulated is a common bipolar symptom. This includes feeling like you can't go on and that you have to quit what you're doing because of the pressure. Feeling overwhelmed in crowds, feeling pressured by others, wanting to hide in bed, wanting to run away, and feeling physically uncomfortable and anxious are other common symptoms. These feelings are often triggered by taking on too much, so lifestyle management is often the key to dealing with them.

THE GOOD NEWS

When symptoms appear to be random and chaotic, with no apparent rhyme or reason, it's easy to feel overwhelmed. It's important that you and everyone around you understand the symptoms listed above and come to see them as common and even predictable manifestations of bipolar disorder. Not only can this take the mystery out of the experience of bipolar disorder episodes, but it can also help you to communicate clearly with your doctor when particular symptoms emerge. Finally, knowing the nature of these symptoms is also a necessary starting point for developing a rational treatment plan.

Your Major Symptoms

After each heading, write the main problems you have under each symptom. Add any other major bipolar disorder symptoms you may experience as well.

Depression: _____

_____

Mania: _____

_____

Psychosis: _____

_____

Anxiety: _____

_____

Irritation, anger, aggression, and violent behavior: _____

_____

_____

■ *For Family and Friends*

Family members and friends can fill in this list as well. You can then compare notes with your loved one.

Cognitive/ADHD symptoms: _____

_____

Obsessive/compulsive symptoms: _____

_____

Overstimulated symptoms: _____

_____

KNOWING THAT YOU'RE IN GOOD COMPANY

"Well, even in that deep misery I felt my energy revive, and I said to myself: In spite of everything I shall rise again, I will take up my pencil, which I have forsaken in great discouragement, and I will go on with my drawing, and from that moment everything has seemed transformed in me."

—Vincent van Gogh

Did you know that the painter Vincent van Gogh had bipolar disorder? He was a classic case of Bipolar I. Naturally, his friends and family asked him questions such as, "What is wrong with you? Why can't you settle down, find a nice woman, get married, and have a real career? Why are you always fighting with people and painting those wild pictures?" Sound familiar? You may know the story of how he cut off his ear. Did you know that he actually only cut off a part of his ear after a very stressful fight (a typical bipolar disorder trigger) with his roommate—the painter Paul Gauguin? He then wrapped up the piece of his ear, took it to a prostitute, handed it to her, and said, "Keep this like a treasure." The local papers thought he was crazy, of course. When this manic/psychotic episode ended, he was just as confused as anyone as to what had happened.

Luckily, he found an amazing doctor, of whom he painted a very famous portrait. Dr. Gachet was a compassionate and loving man, but he had little to work with in the late 1800s. At that time, the only treatment for the illness was rest and talk. No one understood how van Gogh could be so many different people at one time. How could he be so loving to his brother Theo and yet have so many problems with other people? How could he take in a prostitute and her daughter and give them his love and then go into a rage of depression and destroy all of his relationships once again? There were no answers. Finally, after a particularly bad downswing, he took his own life.

Why is this story important for you to know? Because it shows that a man you never met, who lived more than a hundred years ago, had exactly the same symptoms as every other person with bipolar disorder. He had the same struggles, the same issues with his friends and family members, and went through the same questioning and worrying about his life that people with the illness go through today. The illness is just that: an illness that doesn't change. It's nothing personal. It has nothing to do with your personality or your talent, and is not even a reflection on your ability to handle life. The positive news is that you have so many more options than van Gogh had. You have medications, educated doctors, effective treatments, and books designed to help you see that there is hope and you can get better. As you read the rest of this book, continually remind yourself that, like van Gogh, you simply have an illness that needs to be understood and treated like any other illness with specific symptoms. There is nothing wrong with you. And as a family member or friend, you can remember van Gogh when you think your loved one is just being difficult!

KNOWLEDGE MATTERS

Learning about bipolar disorder puts you in control and helps you become a participant in your own healing, instead of just a spectator to the professionals who manage your medications. Knowledge really is power. The more you know, the more likely you are to remind yourself that this is just an illness that needs management, instead of feeling that it's some personal failing on your part because your emotions are all over the place.

Now that you know more about the history of bipolar disorder, its different diagnoses, and its specific and predictable symptoms, you are ready to learn to treat the illness successfully by using the 4-Step Plan. You really do have many options in the treatment of this illness once you learn the basics.

■ *For Family and Friends*

You really do make a difference in the lives of people with bipolar disorder. Family members and friends often play the caretaking role without having the tools they need to help their loved one get better. The more you know about the official symptoms of the illness, the more you can help your loved one.

Your Toolbox

Knowledge about bipolar disorder.

A correct diagnosis.

A list of your major symptoms.

MEDICATIONS AND SUPPLEMENTS

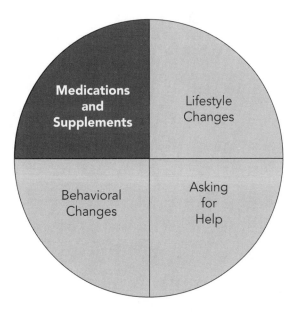

CHAPTER 1

MEDICATIONS AND SUPPLEMENTS

Medications and supplements represent the first section of the treatment plan. This is a difficult and often frustrating part of having bipolar disorder for many people. How many medications are you taking to manage bipolar disorder? Do you sometimes feel overwhelmed with the thought that you will have to take these medications for the rest of your life? Maybe you feel it's unfair. Maybe you have trouble staying on medications because of side effects. Maybe you go through periods in which you pretend that bipolar disorder isn't real and that it will go away if you just ignore it . . . but then you get sick again and have to restart the medications to find stability, and the cycle is repeated.

All of the above behavior is normal. Accepting the bipolar disorder diagnosis is hard enough. Having to accept that you will probably need some form of medication for the rest of your life can be pretty daunting and depressing.

Many, if not most, patients with bipolar disorder experience a significant amount of confusion regarding medical treatment and often receive very little information about the drugs they're taking. Inadequate compliance with medication treatments is the number one reason that there are often negative outcomes for people with bipolar disorder. The goal of this chapter is to offer concise and practical information on the medications currently used to treat bipolar disorder, how they work in your system, and why you need medications in order to stay stable. There is a good reason why this is the first section of the treatment plan: Medications are an essential part of bipolar disorder treatment, and the more you are willing to accept this fact, the better the outcome can be. This chapter does not make light of the significant problems and frustrations people with bipolar disorder have with medications. When you finish this chapter, you will have a clearer idea

■ *For Family and Friends*

As a family member, it may be up to you to help a loved one manage medications, especially if he or she was just diagnosed or is recently out of the hospital. The more you know about the medications used to treat bipolar disorder, the better you can help your loved one. People with bipolar disorder often stop taking their medications, for various and often understandable reasons (for example, because of unpleasant side effects). Appreciating this will give you some perspective when your loved one either goes off medications or refuses to take them. This chapter will give you some tools to help your loved one stay on the medications until he or she finds the right combination with the fewest side effects.

Please note that it's very dangerous for you to encourage your loved one to get off medications and learn to manage the illness alone. It's fine to use supplements and other lifestyle changes to manage bipolar disorder, but to do this without at least some help from medications can be quite difficult and dangerous—especially for people with Bipolar I and serious mania mood swings.

as to why you truly need the medications, and will also have some tips on how to manage these medications so that they treat bipolar disorder instead of taking over your life.

UNDERSTANDING WHAT HAPPENS IN THE BRAIN WHEN YOU'RE SICK

When you're sick, it feels so personal and emotional that it's probably hard for you to remember that being sick simply means that your brain isn't working correctly and needs to be regulated. The goal of bipolar disorder medications is to get your brain back on track so that it can operate more normally and effectively. If you approach medications this way, they may not seem so troublesome and difficult to understand.

The human brain is a tremendously complex organ that carries out two primary roles:

1. Monitoring and regulating the functioning of the body (for example, regulating body temperature, respiration, and hormone levels).
2. Ensuring survival.

Regarding survival, the brain is continuously scanning the environment for potential dangers. It also plans for the future and is in a constant state of readiness to launch adaptive responses. Human beings are capable of remarkable abilities to cope with a host of stressful situations. Like shock absorbers, most people periodically encounter difficult situations, feel the impact, react emotionally, cope to the best of their ability, and then, once the stress is over, bounce back, returning to a less stressful state. Successful coping depends on a number of things, particularly including the ability to think clearly, to problem-solve, and to maintain some measure of emotional control. When episodes occur, people with bipolar disorder lose these faculties and therefore lack the ability to bounce back.

UNDERSTANDING WHY THE BIPOLAR DISORDER BRAIN IS DIFFERENT

The problem is that your brain doesn't always do what it's designed to do. People with bipolar disorder have brains that are less resilient and simply don't respond correctly to the environment. At times, your brain doesn't monitor and regulate the functioning of the body the way it should. Your bipolar brain often creates problems instead of helping you cope with them. Often it simply isn't possible to think clearly, problem-solve, and maintain an appropriate measure of emotional control, because certain brain structures that regulate emotions lose their ability to function appropriately. This appears to be due to abnormal chemical regulation of these brain mechanisms. It can also be caused by actual brain damage, which can begin to gradually occur when people with bipolar disorder either do not get treatment or have poorly controlled, recurrent episodes. What is becoming increasingly clear is that not only do many of the medications used to treat bipolar disorder reduce symptoms and help people maintain emotional stability, but some have what are called neuroprotective properties: They are able to protect the brain from being damaged by the illness, and may actually activate natural mechanisms for the growth of new nerve cells. This has been demonstrated with the mood-stabilizing drug lithium. Lithium promotes the production of a protein, BDNF, which has been shown to activate the birth of new nerve cells in certain areas of the brain (this process is referred to as neurogenesis). Unfortunately, some people view psychiatric medications as a "crutch" that operates only to make or suppress symptoms. Although the drugs do help to control symptoms, in a very real sense they also operate to protect and assist the brain in carrying out certain functions in a more normal and adaptive way (for example, by controlling emotions and mood swings). In much the same way that insulin does not cure diabetes, these drugs do not cure bipolar disorder—but can help normalize biological functioning.

About 30 percent of people who take bipolar disorder medications experience minimal to no side effects, but the truth is that the majority of people do encounter side effects, and often these are considerable. Bipolar disorder medications are often tough to deal with; not only are their side effects difficult to live with, but the medications can also take a number of weeks or even months to start working. However, if you look at the alternative—the fact that a brain with bipolar disorder often has severe functioning limitations—the medications start to look more appealing. It is critical that family members and friends be supportive of these much-needed medications. Getting completely *off* medications should not be your goal, as it almost always leads to disasters. Asking for help in finding the right medications at the right dose is much more realistic.

THE COMPLEX INTERACTION OF BRAIN CHEMICALS

Your ability to adaptively control strong emotions relies on a very complex interaction of brain chemicals operating to regulate the millions of nerve cells in a part of the brain called the limbic system (also commonly referred to as the emotional brain). The limbic system and a closely related brain structure, the hypothalamus, are responsible for igniting appropriate emotional reactions (for example, the fight-or-flight response); for maintaining some degree of control, which is necessary for clear and adaptive thinking; and for getting the brain and body back into a state of homeostasis once the stressful circumstances have subsided. In addition, these brain structures also influence a number of biological functions such as sleep, appetite, sex drive, physical and mental energy, and activity levels.

To carry out these necessary functions, the brain must maintain a delicate balance of neurochemicals—most notably serotonin, norepinephrine, glutamate, GABA, and dopamine. A good analogy is that the brain is like a thermostat in your home. There is a comfort range set on most thermostats. The built-in thermometer in the thermostat is constantly monitoring the temperature in the room. If the temperature rises above a certain point, the air conditioner automatically turns on. If it falls below a particular temperature, the furnace comes on. Such automatic monitoring and fine-tuned adjustments also are constantly at work within the brain, to maintain a relative emotional comfort zone.

Your Thermostat Is Broken

The problem for people with bipolar disorder is that the thermostat in the brain doesn't always do its job correctly. Medical research has clearly documented that bipolar disorder involves a *biologically based* impaired ability to effectively regulate intense emotions—just like a broken thermostat that can't monitor the temperature correctly. There is nothing wrong with you psychologically; instead, there is something wrong with your brain's neurochemistry.

Your Brain Is Very Sensitive

Because your brain doesn't function as a normal brain should, outside events and your own behaviors can lead to serious mood swings. Sleep deprivation or disruption is a notorious trigger for bipolar mood swings, as are other factors that can significantly alter hormonal functioning and brain chemistry. Stressful life events can provoke shifts into overwhelming states of mania or depression. And even in the absence of specific stressors, abnormal neurochemical functioning in the limbic system can, at times, spontaneously provoke the emergence of intense mood swings, like a thermostat that for no apparent reason turns on the furnace, even though the house is already warm. This explains why you can't by willpower alone *just get a handle on your emotions.*

Medications are designed to regulate your emotions and get your brain back on track so that it can respond correctly to life events. It's not the goal of medications to take away your creativity, numb you to the reality of life, or change your personality. They are simply meant to regulate your brain thermostat so that it can work correctly. Understanding and appreciating the biological basis of bipolar disorder is critical for those with the illness and for family members and close friends. As you will read in this book, a number of very effective strategies can help to stabilize and normalize brain chemistry for people suffering from bipolar disorder, and certain psychiatric medications are the most direct and powerful way to accomplish this.

Cortisol: The Stress Hormone

Unless bipolar disorder is well controlled, most people suffering from this illness will spend many, many months in episodes of depression. One very significant health consequence of untreated depression is an extreme elevation of the stress hormone cortisol. Cortisol is normally not at all dangerous to the body, but the exposure to prolonged elevations seen in severe depression is considered to be toxic and to influence general health.

High, sustained levels of cortisol damage the interior walls of blood vessels. This eventually can lead to artery disease and a very significant increased risk of strokes and heart disease. Death rates from heart attacks among people with poorly controlled depression are twice those seen in age-matched adults without bipolar disorder.

High cortisol also has a significant impact on the immune system, resulting in a weakened ability to fight diseases. Rates of death due to infectious diseases are two to three times higher in people experiencing prolonged periods of depression.

Finally, high cortisol levels also reduce the release of growth hormone. This greatly contributes to an increased risk of developing osteoporosis.

Effective medication treatments for bipolar disorder not only target devastating mood swings, but also can contribute significantly to lowering risks for these serious medical disorders.

KNOWING YOUR CURRENT MEDICATION OPTIONS

The choice of medications used to treat bipolar disorder depends on the mood state you're currently experiencing—mania, depression, or another major symptom such as psychosis or anxiety. In addition, medication choices always must take into consideration the ultimate goal of preventing recurrences.

Currently, there are eleven medications approved by the Food and Drug Administration (FDA) for the treatment of bipolar disorder: lithium, Thorazine, Risperdal, Seroquel, Geodon, Abilify, Equetro, Symbyax, Depakote, Lamictal, and Zyprexa. However, a number of other highly effective drugs are in common use. The use of medications not approved by the FDA for the treatment of certain conditions is referred to as off-label use; it must be emphasized that off-label use of medications is very common in every branch of medicine.

Why So Many Pills for One Illness?

Recent surveys reveal that in the United States, only 11 percent of people being treated for bipolar disorder take just a single drug (called monotherapy). On average, most people being treated for bipolar disorder take three or four medications simultaneously. The reason for this is simple: Medication combinations are often necessary to adequately treat the wide array of symptoms seen in this illness.

What to Expect from Medication Treatment

Bipolar disorder is like a number of other chronic medical conditions, such as diabetes, asthma, or arthritis. It's not a condition that can be *cured* by currently available medications. However, the medications discussed later in this chapter are effective in relieving many of the more serious symptoms of bipolar disorder and often can reduce the frequency of mood episodes for most people, if they receive appropriate treatment.

With aggressive, appropriate, and ongoing medication treatment, which is started during the first or second mood episode, about 30 percent of people do not experience *severe* recurrences.[1] Thus, in about one out of five people, the medications are highly successful in preventing significant relapses (as long as people continue to take them). This of course leads to the question: What about the other 80 percent of people with bipolar disorder, especially those who go through many episodes before being adequately diagnosed and treated? The facts are that when people do *not* receive effective medication treatment during the first several episodes of bipolar disorder or are given the wrong medications because they have been misdiagnosed, medication outcomes are not as positive as they are for those who receive the correct treatment during the first episode. Certainly in the case of people who are diagnosed later than the first or second episode, many people do respond to medication treatments, but delays in getting treatment can make it more challenging to successfully control the disorder. Still, people can find significant relief. Even after starting medication treatment after the first or second mood swing, the recurrence rates for *severe* episodes can be reduced by about 75 percent, and hospitalizations can often be avoided when the correct medications are used. Subsequent episodes that do

Hazel's Story

Age 46

I've never seen anything like the difference in my daughter since she started medications. She was manic from the time she was sixteen. In fact she was out of control and living on the streets for a while. She got in trouble with drugs and when
the police found her purse on the roof of a drug house, they found her and took
her to the station for questioning. It was the best thing that ever happened to her.
She was clearly manic and they put her in seventy-two-hour observation where she
received medications and took them for the first time in her life. About the third
week she was there, I walked in and she said, "Hi, Mom." And I could tell I had
my daughter back. It was like someone was in her body for all of those years. I know
it's an illness and it was never her fault, but I get so angry for the lost years. Then I
remind myself that she's back. I think she was just finally old enough to see where
her life would be without medications. She works now and has a family. She still
gets mood swings, but they are nothing like they were before medications—we can
deal with them as a family now that we have a treatment plan for the tough times.

occur tend to be milder (as opposed to severe) depressions and hypomanias.[2] These statistics show that medications work in preventing serious bipolar disorder relapses, but they
are far from perfect. And, as mentioned in this chapter, it may take quite awhile to find
the right combination.

BIPOLAR DISORDER MEDICATIONS: AN OVERVIEW

The following section will help you as well as your family members and friends understand
the different types of medications used to treat bipolar disorder. Please note that this chapter
includes only a general outline of current bipolar disorder medications. It's suggested that
you always research any medication that your doctor suggests at your local library and online. You need to know the dosage guidelines, potential drug interactions, and any other information that's important to you personally. Taking a drug blindly can lead to problems.

> ### *Being an Informed Consumer*
>
> Do you know:
>
> - What drugs you're taking?
> - The specific symptoms they're treating?
> - The recommended dosage?
> - Any potential interactions?
> - Their side effects?
>
> Talk with your doctor, research the drugs in books and on the Internet, and talk with your pharmacist so that you can ask intelligent and informed questions when you go to your appointments.

It's a good idea for you to ask your doctor any questions you may have about your medications, and the more information you already have, the easier it will be to talk with your doctor. You want to be an informed patient. It helps if family members are also well informed.

There are six categories of psychiatric medications that have been found to be effective in treating bipolar disorder:

1. Lithium.
2. Anticonvulsants.
3. Antipsychotics.
4. Antidepressants (including Symbyax, which is a combination of an antidepressant and an antipsychotic—Prozac and Zyprexa).
5. Calcium channel blockers.
6. Benzodiazepines (tranquilizers).

The following table gives you some examples from the preceding categories. Notice that the drugs are known by a generic name and one or more brand names, and that dosages differ greatly depending on the drug. It's always suggested that you research every drug you are taking or might take, so that you are aware of the generally agreed-upon dosage ranges, the potential side effects, and what food and drugs you need to avoid while taking the drug.

There is a chart in appendix C you can use to track your medications.

MEDICATIONS

	Generic Name	Brand Name	Suggested Daily Dosage
Mood stabilizers			
	lithium	Eskalith, Lithonate	600–2400 mg
Anticonvulsants			
	divalproex	Depakote	750–1500 mg
	carbamazepine	Tegretol	600–1600 mg
	oxcarbazepine	Trileptal	1200–2400 mg
	lamotrigine	Lamictal	50–500 mg
	topiramate	Topamax	50–300 mg
	gabapentin	Neurontin	300–2400 mg

Atypical antipsychotics (newly developed antipsychotic medications that treat psychotic symptoms and appear to have antimanic effects)

	Generic Name	Brand Name	Suggested Daily Dosage
	olanzapine	Zyprexa	5–20 mg
	risperidone	Risperdal	2–16 mg
	ziprasidone	Geodon	60–160 mg
	aripiprazole	Abilify	15–30 mg
	quetiapine	Seroquel	150–400 mg

Antidepressants

	Generic Name	Brand Name	Suggested Daily Dosage
	fluoxetine	Prozac, Sarafem	20–80 mg
	bupropion	Wellbutrin	150–400 mg
	sertraline	Zoloft	50–200 mg
	paroxetine	Paxil	20–50 mg
	venlafaxine	Effexor	75–350 mg
	nefazodone	Serzone	100–500 mg
	mirtazapine	Remeron	15–45 mg
	citalopram	Celexa	10–60 mg
	escitalopram	Lexapro	5–20 mg
	duloxetine	Cymbalta	20–80 mg
	atomoxepine	Strattera	60–120 mg

*Calcium channel blockers**

	Generic Name	Brand Name	Suggested Daily Dosage
	verapamil	Calan, Isoptin	360–480 mg

Benzodiazepines (also referred to as minor tranquilizers or antianxiety drugs)

	Generic Name	Brand Name	Suggested Daily Dosage
	diazepam	Valium	4–30 mg
	clonazepam	Klonopin	0.5–2 mg
	lorazepam	Ativan	1–6 mg
	alprazolam	Xanax	1–4 mg

MEDICATIONS   *(continued)*

	Generic Name	Brand Name	Suggested Daily Dosage
Benzodiazepine sleeping pills			
	temazepam	Restoril	15–30 mg
	triazolam	Halcion	0.25–0.5 mg
	zolpidem	Ambien	5–10 mg
	zaleplon	Sonata	5–10 mg
	eszopiclone	Lunesta	1–3 mg

*When a nerve impulse occurs, channels open up at the end of certain nerve cells, allowing calcium to enter. The calcium influx helps to release the neurotransmitter from the vesicles (where it's stored). Thus, blocking calcium channels slows the rate of nerve-cell firing. These drugs were developed to treat heart conditions but have been found to be effective in treating mania.

Be Careful!

- Some anticonvulsant mood stabilizers and lithium have been associated with causing birth defects. Talk with your doctor if you're pregnant or planning to get pregnant and are taking these drugs.
- Tegretol, Trileptal, Topamax, and the herb St.-John's-wort can interfere with the actions of birth control pills.
- All benzodiazepines are potentially habit forming and can be addicting if taken by people who have a history of drug addictions or alcoholism.
- Neurontin (generic name gabapentin) is a non-habit-forming alternative to benzodiazepines that can reduce anxiety but without risk of addiction. Recent studies have shown Neurontin to be ineffective in treating mania, but it's often added to other mood stabilizers because of its ability to reduce anxiety.

MORE INFORMATION ON ANTIDEPRESSANT MEDICATIONS

There is currently some controversy regarding the use of antidepressants in the treatment of bipolar disorder depression. Antidepressants were first developed in the 1950s and have a solid track record of success in the treatment of unipolar depression. (Unipolar is the more common variety of depression, which affects up to 17 percent of people in the United States.[3]) But their use in bipolar disorder has some limitations:

- Large-scale studies looking at treatment outcomes for hundreds of patients appear to indicate that antidepressants alone (as monotherapy) are not significantly more effective than placebos in treating bipolar depression. However, as important as group studies are, they fail to highlight that *some* individuals do, in fact, appear to respond to antidepressants. The point is, the research suggests that, *in general,* the effectiveness of antidepressants alone is not robust.
- Antidepressants can, at times, cause what is known as a switch. When this occurs, it's typically seen during the first two to three weeks of treatment with antidepressants. The person rather rapidly comes out of the depression and goes into a state of mania or hypomania. *This is a serious treatment complication.*
- Some evidence indicates that the use of antidepressants (especially over a prolonged period of time) *may* cause a condition referred to as cycle acceleration. This is an overall worsening of the illness in which major mood episodes become more frequent and more severe. This is also a serious treatment complication.
- All antidepressants studied have shown that between 3 and 4 percent of people starting treatment experience increased thoughts about suicide. This generally occurs either in the first two weeks of treatment (before the medication effects kick in) or after discontinuing the medication. Many of the antidepressants can cause some initial "activation," or restlessness, as a side effect, and this can be experienced a few hours after the first dose. In seriously depressed people, this restlessness can add to the sense of discomfort and may be why some people experience the increase in suicidal thoughts. This is a real issue, although it affects a small percentage of patients. *If this happens to you, contact your doctor as soon as possible.* Often other medications such as tranquilizers can be prescribed to reduce the restlessness until the antidepressant begins to take effect. Also, always report any suicidal feeling to your doctor. These thoughts should be taken seriously.

There is general agreement that these potential problems with antidepressants do exist, but the fact remains that some individual patients do have a positive response to antidepressants. Recent studies reveal that despite these risks, 19 percent of people experiencing bipolar depression must have antidepressants added to mood stabilizers in order to achieve successful resolution of their depressions. We must be very clear that antidepressants are not recommended as a monotherapy—in other words, they should never be taken alone—and must be taken along with a mood stabilizer. It's important that you talk with your doctor about these issues.

OVER-THE-COUNTER SUPPLEMENTS

Billions of dollars each year are spent on over-the-counter dietary supplements and herbal products. Obviously, many people seek out this kind of treatment, and studies have shown that 70 percent of people taking these supplements never mention them to their doctors. Some of the top sellers are products that claim to have an impact on emotions and brain functioning, including St.-John's-wort and SAM-e. These two over-the-counter drugs do, in fact, have a significant amount of research documenting their effectiveness in treating some forms of depression. To date, however, they have not been adequately studied in the treatment of bipolar disorder. What is clear is that any drug—prescription or over-the-counter—that reduces depression can actually trigger mania in someone with bipolar disorder. This fact has been well documented in the cases of St.-John's-wort and SAM-e, and thus neither should ever be taken except under careful monitoring by a psychiatrist. In addition, St.-John's-wort has been shown to have very significant drug interactions when taken by people also taking other prescription medications. Such interactions can be potentially dangerous. Never take either of these over-the-counter products without consulting your physician.

Omega-3 Fatty Acids

One exception to the research on over-the-counter supplements and bipolar disorder is the use of omega-3 fatty acids. Omega-3 fatty acids are an essential ingredient in brain structure and functioning: 30 to 35 percent of the brain mass is made up of these fatty acids. Several research studies have shown omega-3 fatty acid supplements to be a helpful adjunct in stabilizing mood in bipolar disorder[4] and, more recently, in the treatment of unipolar depression.[5] Initially, large doses were tried (9 grams per day), but more recent studies suggest that 1 to 2 grams (1000 to 2000 mg) a day may be as effective with fewer side effects. Omega-3 fatty acids generally are available in 0.5-gram (500 mg) or 1-gram (1000 mg) capsules. It is definitely beneficial for you to talk with your health care professional about omega-3 fatty acids.

Problems and Solutions for Over-the-Counter Supplements

There are three potentially very serious problems when it comes to the use of over-the-counter products:

- The Food and Drug Administration doesn't regulate the production of such dietary supplements. In other words, you can never be sure if the product contains the ingredients listed on the label. Some over-the-counter products have been found to have inadequate amounts of the mood-altering ingredient or to contain contaminants.
- As noted above, some of these over-the-counter products can cause very significant drug interactions. Most notably, a large number of people have experienced serious drug interactions while taking St.-John's-wort with other medications. Keep in mind that "natural" does not necessarily mean "safe." At times, drug interactions can actually kill you.
- Anything that reduces depression can potentially provoke a manic episode in people with bipolar disorder. SAM-e and St.-John's-wort have both done this.

Despite the aforementioned cautions, some people do, in fact, benefit from some over-the-counter supplements for treating mood symptoms or for reducing side effects. Here are some guidelines for exploring your options safely.

- Always talk with your doctor before introducing supplements.
- See a qualified naturopathic doctor who has experience treating bipolar disorder to talk about your supplemental options.
- Talk with a pharmacist about potential interactions between bipolar disorder medications and over-the-counter products.
- Look for a label that says USP (US Pharmacopoeia) or NDF (National Sanitation Foundation). These labels let you know that the product has been independently

tested to verify that it contains the ingredients listed and is free from contaminants. This doesn't necessarily mean that the product is effective, but it does let you know the bottle contains what it says it does.

TRACKING YOUR MEDICATIONS AND SUPPLEMENTS

When introducing new medications and supplements, especially if you are taking more than one, it's imperative that you keep a record of what you're taking, the dosage, and when you take the medications. There is a chart in appendix C called "Track Your Medications." This record can be invaluable for both you and your doctors as you create your comprehensive treatment plan. It will help you to remember your dosage and the different medications and supplements you have tried. There is also a section in which you can chart your side effects and write any questions you may have for your next doctor's visit. Remember, many people take up to a year or more to find the right medication combinations. If you're in the first few months of treatment, give yourself time for you and your doctor to get it right, but be vigilant about charting your medications, your supplements, and their side effects.

You may be taking one drug from each category mentioned earlier in the chapter; this is normal, especially in the first stages of treating the illness. For many people, some of these drugs can be reduced or eliminated as the current episode subsides and more effective management skills are mastered. In every case, however, it's essential that you know what medications you're putting in your body. You should be able to answer the following questions about each medication you take:

- What is the normal dose?
- When should I take the medications?
- What are the side effects?
- Are there any potential drug interactions?
- Do I need any lab tests?
- How long does the drug normally take to work?
- Are there special foods I need to avoid?

Your health care provider, the library, and the Internet are good resources for answering these questions. A family member or friend can also be a great help if you're just too worn out to do a lot of research.

WHAT TO DO IF YOUR FIRST MEDICATIONS DON'T WORK

It's normal if you have to try a few medications before you find the right combination—the one that helps you find stability. It can take some time to see what medications will work for your specific biological makeup. You must anticipate that it is *extremely common* for doctors to make initial medication choices, begin treatment, and then, during the following weeks or months, make what are often frequent changes in the doses or medications prescribed. You or your family members may become worried as you begin to encounter side effects or experience what seems like an endless number of lab tests or changes in medications or doses. Many people become concerned that such changes suggest that their doctor may not be competent, or that their case of bipolar disorder is especially treatment-resistant. These worries can lead to discouragement and pessimism.

The reality is that the pathway to recovery and good outcomes, more often than not, is complicated. The *rule,* not the exception, is trying several (often many) medications in the search for just the right drug or combination. Frequent changes in medications are not necessarily a reason for concern. While it's important to be informed and not to just try medication after medication without questioning your health care professional, the fact is that bipolar disorder is challenging to treat, and systematically trying various medications in the search for the right combination is a time-consuming process.

WHY YOU NEED TO TAKE YOUR MEDICATIONS
EVEN WHEN YOU FEEL WELL

Taking medications when you feel well flies in the face of common sense. You must remember, however, that bipolar disorder is recurring, and over a period of time there is a tendency for episodes to become increasingly severe and harder to treat. And as noted earlier, some research indicates that untreated or poorly treated bipolar disorder can ultimately result in lasting damage to the nervous system, while ongoing treatment with bipolar medications may prevent this.

What to Do If You're Thinking of Stopping Your Medications

First of all, it's important to know that one very common symptom of bipolar disorder, especially in mania or hypomania, is poor insight. This is an inaccurate awareness of the need to stay on medications. And this is often understandable in the early stages of a manic episode since people may feel very happy and upbeat. It's a catch-22, because the best way to prevent severe episodes is to stay on your medications and yet the thoughts created by the illness itself can tell you that you don't really need medications. Medication treatments are far from perfect, but they offer the kind of effectiveness that can substantially reduce suffering, keep families together, avoid catastrophes, and save lives.

Unfortunately, the facts show that there's a good chance that there will come a time when you will want to stop your medications. What can you do to prevent this? Some tips include using this book to significantly reduce your symptoms so that you may, in the long run, be able to take fewer medications or lower doses (always with your doctor's supervision). You should also constantly remind yourself what life is like for you when you don't take medications and ask for help from your loved ones in maintaining your medications. And finally, simply stopping your medications can lead to some very serious withdrawal symptoms including suicidal thoughts and extreme physical discomfort. The checklist on pages 50 and 51 can help remind you of why you need medications to treat bipolar disorder.

■ *For Family and Friends*

If your loved one does stop his or her medications, you may feel scared, incredulous, angry, and frustrated. Unfortunately, this is a very normal part of bipolar disorder. Side effects can become too strong to live with; the illness itself can also tell people that they are fine and don't need medications. If you had been depressed for months and then suddenly felt better, wouldn't you want to get off the medications? It's normal that people with mania feel that the illness is cured. And although it's often dangerous and destructive, it's very normal for people to go off and on medications until they find the right combination.

Anyone who suspects that loved ones are ready to stop or want to stop medications should have them read this section again. They do have options. Going off medications can be catastrophic both for them and for the people in their lives. Remind them that they can change medications, try microdosing (explained later in the chapter), and use the tips in this book to reduce their symptoms and hopefully reduce their need for medications. Going off medications is not really an option, especially for those with troubling mania or suicidal thoughts.

Look over the following lists and check the entries that are true for you. You will probably have a few positive experiences when off medications, but the point of this exercise is to see that the bad outweighs the supposed good.

Life Before Medications

- ☐ Relationship problems.
- ☐ Lots of crying.
- ☐ Unhappiness.
- ☐ Recklessness.
- ☐ Restlessness/craving constant change.
- ☐ Spending issues.
- ☐ Inability to work effectively.
- ☐ Bombardment with too many ideas.
- ☐ Dangerous behavior.
- ☐ Inability to know how you really feel.
- ☐ Constantly feeling up and down.
- ☐ Feeling misunderstood.
- ☐ Inability to stay in one place or stick with anything.
- ☐ Racing thoughts that don't stop.
- ☐ Constant irritability.
- ☐ Expanded creativity.
- ☐ Excessive anxiousness.
- ☐ Ability to work abnormally long hours when manic.

Life After Medications

- ☐ Greater stability.
- ☐ Fewer worries.
- ☐ Better able to connect with people.
- ☐ Ability to work and support yourself.
- ☐ Worrying about being dulled by medications.
- ☐ Ability to live life again.
- ☐ Less anxiety.
- ☐ No longer hearing voices.
- ☐ Worrying about being less creative.
- ☐ Ability to think about one thing at a time.

☐ Being told that others find it easier to be around you.
☐ Wondering if this is the "real you."
☐ Wondering if the medications are changing your personality.
☐ Less destructive behavior—for instance, drinking less.

It helps if you look at the alternatives before you make the decision to stop your medications. The remainder of this chapter gives you more ideas on how to reduce side effects and find alternatives to stopping your medications.

THE REALITY OF SIDE EFFECTS

All medications have side effects, and, unfortunately, the drugs used to treat bipolar disorder are known to produce side effects for the majority of people taking them. Side effects are at times mild and easy to tolerate. But often they are more noticeable, and in rare instances they can be dangerous.

When people take medications for any medical condition, the drugs enter the circulation and travel to every cell in the body. Drug companies have attempted to develop medications that pinpoint their actions in certain parts of the nervous system while having little impact on other bodily tissues, but the reality is that many bipolar disorder medications affect the whole body. To date, there have been some improvements (especially with the newer antidepressants and antipsychotics), but we still have a long way to go. You can't harpoon a drug into the brain and keep it there. The drug molecules go everywhere. Many bodily tissues are responsive to the same molecules that are active in the nervous system. One notable example is that a number of antidepressants and mood stabilizers increase the amount of the neurotransmitter serotonin. This action may account for the antidepressant action in the brain. However, more than 90 percent of serotonin-responsive cells reside in the gut. Thus, a lot of people develop gastrointestinal side effects such as nausea, diarrhea, and gas when they take these medications.

It's well documented that even when a current episode has subsided, people with bipolar disorder *must* continue to take medications in order to prevent or reduce the likelihood of recurrence. Unfortunately, up to 90 percent of people who start treatment for their first bipolar disorder episode will recover from this episode but, within weeks or months, will simply stop taking their medications, against medical advice.

The most common reasons for doing so are understandable:

■ Problematic side effects. Many people start to think, *Why should I stay on the pills if my episode is over and all the pills seem to do is cause side effects?*

■ In addition, many people conclude that the episode they experienced was not really bipolar disorder but just an unfortunate single episode that won't recur.[6] It's hard to accept a lifelong illness, and people can and will often talk themselves out of taking the medications, even when the symptoms return almost immediately.

Once again, these reasons are understandable, but they almost invariably lead to the emergence of more episodes. What does this information mean to you? Statistics can seem remote, but if up to 90 percent of people with bipolar disorder tend to go off med-

■ *For Family and Friends*

How can you as a family member or friend help with side effects? The first step is education about the drugs your loved one is taking. Can you list them? What is each one for? What are its specific side effects? It also helps if you understand that the drugs that help the brain can absolutely wreck the body. Problems can range from weight gain and hair loss to muscle and dental issues. If your loved one had cancer and went through chemotherapy (often defined as the use of chemical agents to treat or control disease), you would certainly understand the physical side effects of the drugs. You would expect hair loss, vomiting, diarrhea, muscle pain, vision problems, shaking, excessive tiredness, weight issues, sleep disturbances, and more. And yet when a person with bipolar disorder takes drugs, the side effects are often downplayed by family members and friends. "Why don't you just take your medications like you should? Don't you want to be stable? What are you thinking? The side effects can't be that bad." The reality is that the side effects *can* be that bad, which is why it's so important that people with bipolar disorder find the correct drugs at the right dose. Bipolar disorder medications affect brain chemicals, and the brain controls the function of the body. These drugs are serious, and you need to take them seriously if you want to help your loved one.

ications, it's time for you to take note. Unless you have a plan in place to prevent this behavior in yourself, there's a good chance you will do the same.

Managing Side Effects

The good news is that many side effects can be managed by dosage adjustments or by switching to other medications. This is one reason that most people will need to go through trials on a variety of medications to determine which ones are the most effective and best tolerated. It's also important for you to know as much as possible about the medications you're prescribed. Family members need to be in on this process, too, because they are often the ones who help the person with bipolar disorder deal with side effects. In the past, doctors prescribed medications and patients quietly complied, but times have changed—for the better. These days, more and more people have become informed consumers. There is a lot you can do to learn about current medication treatments (the pros and the cons), and you have a perfect right to ask any and all questions you may have about medications prescribed. The more that people are actively engaged as collaborators with their doctor, the better treatment outcomes become. In other words, don't be scared to talk with your doctor about your medication issues, including the desire to stop medications.

Unfortunately, some people have had the experience of speaking with a physician and asking questions, only to encounter defensiveness, impatience, or resistance. Clearly this does happen, but appropriate medical treatment requires open lines of communication between the patient and the doctor. Openness to legitimate questions is also a compassionate way of treating fellow human beings, especially those struggling with bipolar disorder. If you cannot successfully speak with your doctor due to his or her own defensiveness, then maybe it's time to find a more open-minded physician.

Every effort should be made to find the right medication or medication combination in an attempt to minimize side effects. And often this can be accomplished. Still, many people simply end up having to tolerate some side effects; it's not pleasant, but it's ultimately necessary to reduce or eliminate severe mood swings. And, unfortunately, a very small number of people are just unable to tolerate any current bipolar disorder medications at all. (If this describes you, don't give up hope. You can continue to work with your doctor, use the tips in this book to stay stable, and keep trying new medications as they are released on the market.)

Talking with Your Doctor About Side Effects

There is always a time period before drugs begin working. This can range from days to weeks to months, so it's important that you know when to expect a drug to start helping your symptoms. You can research this information and then talk with your doctor about your concerns, especially if you feel the dose is too high or too low.

As the weeks go by on a new medication, you may experience some symptom improvement, but if it's not dramatic or if you're having trouble with noticeable side effects, it's natural that you will want to talk with your doctor about changing medications. Many times you will be told to just stay with the medication, giving it enough time to work. There often is a good reason for this—many people do benefit if they stay on medications long enough for the clinical effect to kick in. Although some symptom changes may be seen within the first week, true resolution of mood episodes takes a long time. This may be discouraging, but you need to know what to expect. A recent study conducted by the National Institute of Mental Health indicates that, on average, it takes ten to twelve weeks to recover from a manic episode, nineteen weeks for a depressive episode, and up to thirty-six weeks to recover from mixed mania.[7] It must be emphasized that substantial reduction in painful emotional symptoms often occurs much earlier than these time frames indicate, but true recovery simply takes a long time.

Many people encounter a combination of unpleasant side effects and a lack of quick response. While it's understandable that this can lead to discouragement, those who stop taking the medication against medical advice often get sicker, ultimately having to start all over again.

Taking charge of your own treatment while still remaining reasonable is essential and will help you communicate with your doctor. You have to decide what you can and can't tolerate in terms of side effects. There's a fine line between what's considered normal for side effects and what's unacceptable. If you're sleeping fourteen hours a day and have gained forty pounds, then it's time for you to talk with your doctor. If you can't live your life because of a certain specific side effect, such as a respiratory problem or a serious rash, it's time to talk with your doctor. This may be difficult—as it's often hard to get an appointment and may be quite intimidating to stick up for yourself—but it has to be done, especially if you're thinking of missing doses or stopping your medications.

The following suggestions can help you to talk with your doctor about medications:

- Can you please tell me why I'm on this particular medication?
- I know that it's important that I stay on medications and I'm willing to do that, but these side effects are simply too strong for me right now. I can't function normally if I am sleeping all day or constantly running to the bathroom because of diarrhea. What are my options?
- How long do you think I need to wait to see results from this medication, and what if I can't wait that long?
- What ideas do you have for reducing side effects?
- Are there any new medications coming out that will work with fewer side effects?
- I could really use help with this. Do you have any suggestions on where I can find more help?

If you're at that place where you're unwilling to stick with your medications, you must find a way to effectively communicate your feelings to your doctor by saying something along the lines of the following: "I understand that your recommendation is to just keep taking the medication. I believe that it's important for me to be able to be open and honest with you about my treatment. I need you to know that I'm at a point where I'm probably just going to stop the medication on my own, and I'd like to ask you to please consider other options. Would you be willing to let me know other medication choices that you think might be an alternative to what I'm currently taking?"

Dealing with side effects is a large part of living with this illness. When you're on a combination of drugs, it makes sense that you would encounter a combination of side effects. Look over the following list and see if you have experienced any of the listed side effects. Put a check mark next to those you're experiencing now and share this information with your doctor.

- ☐ Tiredness and fatigue.
- ☐ Weight gain.
- ☐ Tremors and shakiness.
- ☐ Nausea or diarrhea.
- ☐ Rashes.
- ☐ Memory problems.
- ☐ Menstrual irregularities.
- ☐ Rapid cycling.

- ☐ Suicidal thoughts.
- ☐ Irritability or anger.
- ☐ What seems like a bottomless pit of hunger.
- ☐ No appetite at all.
- ☐ Excessive sleeping.
- ☐ Agitated sleep.
- ☐ Trouble concentrating.
- ☐ Hair loss.
- ☐ Teeth problems.
- ☐ Skin problems.
- ☐ Vision problems.
- ☐ Muscle fatigue.
- ☐ Increased thirst and urination (with lithium).
- ☐ Trouble reading or writing.

Many of these side effects can be quite debilitating if they're allowed to continue. Of course, there are some side effects you simply have to live with in order to stay stable, such as a dry mouth or milder versions of the issues listed above. You're the one who decides when the side effects become too difficult to manage. The point of this section is to remind you that there are steps you can take to get help with these problems. Stopping your medications does not have to be the first step. Doing your own research and then asking for help with medication management is an option.

Here are some more tips for managing side effects:

- Talk about reducing the dose or changing medications with your doctor. Be honest about how you feel and ask for help. If you're thinking of stopping the medications, explain why.
- Work on the things you can change by using the ideas in this book to reduce bipolar disorder symptoms, so that you may need fewer medications or a lower dosage.
- Use the diet and exercise tips in chapter 2 to help you reduce side effects including weight gain and strengthen your body so that it can accept the medications.
- Learn your triggers (covered in chapter 4) so that you can reduce your need for medications.
- Learn about new drugs, their side effects, and how they work; ask to try them, if appropriate.

Amanda's Story

Age 31

It took me years to find the correct combination of medications and lifestyle changes. When I was first diagnosed, I remember thinking, *Everything's going to be fine now. All it takes is the right medications and I can get back to my life. I can do my job well. My relationships will get better. I'm a changed woman!* It didn't work. I was on a roller coaster of medications for two years and gained fifty pounds, lost my hair, and was even more depressed. My doctors kept saying to me, "Just wait. You'll find something that works." I believed them. I had made a lot of lifestyle changes during the years I was on medications. But they just were not enough to give me the quality of life I needed. I was always hoping for a miracle—that one day I would just take this magic pill and the bipolar disorder would go away. With my doctor's help, I decided to try a new mood stabilizer. I was not very hopeful. As every month went by, I kept thinking, *This is pointless. I'm never going to find relief from medications. I'll always have these side effects.* Then, after five months of starting with a really small amount and then increasing the dose to the right level, the drug started to work. I got more used to the side effects. Many of them went away after about five more months. For the first time in my life I remember lying in bed with an empty brain, something that I don't think anyone who doesn't have bipolar disorder can understand. It really did feel like a miracle. I have to admit that the drug doesn't take care of everything. In fact, it really only takes care of about 50 percent of my symptoms. But I'll take the 50 percent. It works for me because I use my treatment plan to take care of the other 50 percent. I wish the medications were the only thing I needed. It takes a lot of time to manage this illness, but I know without the medications it would take all my time, and I'm thankful I was patient and gave the drugs a chance to start working. I wish the bipolar disorder would just go away and that I didn't have to worry about medications and watching what I eat and taking care of myself so vigilantly. But I feel the burden is less now that I have a medication that helps.

■ *For Family and Friends*

If you see your loved one having considerable trouble because of side effects—significant weight gain, shuffling instead of walking, drooling during sleep, sleeping all day, getting much more irritated than normal, experiencing suicidal thoughts, or experiencing a lot of physical problems such as teeth pain and hair loss—it is fine to contact his or her doctor yourself if your loved one is not able to do so. (It's also acceptable for you to take part in your loved one's treatment if he or she *is* well enough to do it.) Side effects are a reality with these drugs, but excessive side effects where the person is no longer functioning normally are not acceptable.

This may be difficult, because too many health care professionals ignore family members and certainly do not understand the role a friend can play. Your loved one may be too drugged to function. Maybe you have a son or a roommate who is a zombie from overmedication. This is simply not okay, and there needs to be an intervention from family and friends to get the person with bipolar disorder critical help. Your intervention should be well researched and methodical. You may have to wait a few months for the drugs to work and the side effects to calm down, but if they don't you have the right to get help for your loved one. In contacting your loved one's health care professional, it may be helpful to say something like this: "My [son, friend, partner, husband, what have you] is so drugged he no longer functions normally. I know this is considered better than being manic and out of control (or depressed and suicidal), but lying around all day is not acceptable. I would like to work with you to find the best medication combination that can help my loved one stay stable and have a normally functioning life."

Contacting a loved one's doctor with your concerns must be done delicately, but it can help you find a balance and help your loved one—especially in the case of a young child.

Please note: Family members and friends must check state laws to find out how much access they have to their loved one's treatment plan, medical records, medications, and diagnosis.

What Is Microdosing?

Microdosing may be helpful for people who can't tolerate the side effects on a normal dose of medications. Microdosing works on the concept that those who experience excessive side effects do not metabolize medications as quickly as other people. This means that with even low doses, they encounter high blood levels of the drug and then significant side effects. One solution is to try minute doses of the medications in order to find the balance between effective help and minimum side effects. As a drug is tolerated and the body becomes accustomed to it, it can be very gradually increased. Talk with your doctor about microdosing if you have trouble with side effects.

- Work with a naturopath familiar with bipolar disorder and ask for help with the medication side effects.
- Focus on how the medications help you.
- Know that self-medicating with alcohol or other recreational drugs will always affect the way your body accepts the medications. Ongoing alcohol or other recreational drug use and abuse is one of the most common factors leading to poor treatment outcome. You must take this issue very seriously.
- Talk with your doctor about a concept referred to as microdosing. This is a strategy for people who are very sensitive to medication side effects in which medications are started in tiny doses and very gradually increased until they reach a therapeutic level. This can really make a difference if you have a lot of trouble with side effects.
- There may come a time that you will have to accept certain side effects if it means staying stable.

LETTING GO

It's hard to let go of some of the "good" things about bipolar disorder. Family members are often the ones who see your behavior realistically while you are just looking for a way to feel good again. Maybe you feel that depression is a natural state since the world is a stressful place, and by treating the depression with medications you won't be as sensitive as a friend or partner. Or maybe you miss the creative highs of the first stages of mania. It's easy to get addicted to your own bipolar disorder behavior. The best way to deal with this is to look at the whole picture rationally. Is the creative high you get while manic worth maxing out your credit cards, driving dangerously, taking a trip without telling anyone where you're going, or losing the respect of others because of your wild and erratic behavior? Is the poetry or music you write when depressed worth the risk of not being able to feel love for yourself or others, a lack of sexual desire, or the possibility of suicide? How does your bipolar disorder behavior affect the people in your life or your ability to work and support yourself?

All of these questions have to be asked before you even think of stopping medications and try to treat the illness naturally. When you look at the consequences of untreated bipolar disorder, the medications are worth it. It can be hard to find the real you after you get a bipolar disorder diagnosis and start medications, but if you give it time, the real you can emerge; you'll see that many of the things you did while sick were actually bipolar-disorder-influenced and didn't represent the real you, anyway. Nostalgia for mania can be especially hard to break, but the more you learn to live a normal and stable life, the easier it can be to let go of the past.

ACCEPTANCE

Once you accept that you have an illness that needs medical treatment, accepting medications can get easier. One reason acceptance is difficult for many people is that bipolar disorder doesn't have obvious physical symptoms—it's much easier to treat a broken leg or a nonfunctioning kidney than it is to fix an ill brain. It's essential that your doctor is someone who will work with you until you find the right combinations of medications. If you can let go and not fight the reality of medications, you have a better chance of finding what works for you. This is hard and it may take some time, but making the decision to change is the first step. Instead of being unrealistic and saying, "My goal is to beat this illness and never take medications again," it may be better to say, "My goal is to manage this illness effectively so that I can find medications that work in smaller doses with limited side effects." This is a realistic and reachable goal, and you can do it. People with bipolar disorder can work with family members and friends for support. Working as a team can really make a difference.

DON'T GIVE UP ON MEDICATIONS

The first step of the Take Charge 4-Step Treatment Plan encourages you to really explore all of your medications choices for bipolar disorder. It may take you a long time to find the right medication, but when you do, it can be like having a new life. Keep trying until you find the medication that helps you reduce your symptoms so that you can use the ideas in the rest of the book to truly find stability.

Your Toolbox

Knowledge about bipolar disorder.

A correct diagnosis.

A list of your major symptoms.

Medication knowledge.

Help with side effects.

LIFESTYLE CHANGES

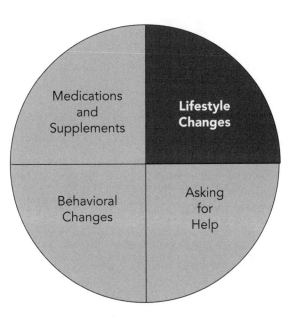

CHAPTER 2

SLEEP, DIET, EXERCISE, AND LIGHT

This chapter introduces you to many important lifestyle changes you can make in addition to your medications. Current medical treatment for bipolar disorder, especially if done in a primary care setting, often minimizes the connections among sleep, diet, exercise, bright light exposure (the intensity of light that you experience outdoors), and other lifestyle choices in treating bipolar disorder in favor of focusing almost exclusively on medications. And yet as you saw in the original description of the treatment plan, these areas are an integral part of any bipolar disorder treatment. Your doctor may be so busy helping you get stable through medications that he or she doesn't have time to explain the ways you can use more natural treatments to maintain stability. Though medications are a very important part of your comprehensive treatment plan, what you do at home is often just as vital.

The key to fostering optimal brain functioning has to do with *environmental* stability. Bipolar disorder brains do not readily adapt to changes in certain physical experiences or stressors even when a person is on medications. Because of this, sleep, diet, exercise, and light do make a significant difference in bipolar disorder. In addition, it makes sense that if you're healthier physically, you will be healthier mentally. Sleep schedules, diet changes, regular exercise, and appropriate bright light exposure can have a direct effect on brain chemistry, in some ways similar to the effects of psychiatric medications.

This chapter offers tips on how to incorporate these healthy lifestyle changes into your new treatment plan. The goal of the chapter is to help you get enough light and exercise, eat a bipolar-friendly diet, and create a regular sleep schedule in order to create neurochemical stability. This chapter is not about rejecting medications, but instead about using more natural methods to control mood swings that *in combination with* medical treatment may at some point reduce symptoms enough to enable you to use lower doses of medications and thus reduce side effects. Another bonus is that most of the suggestions in this chapter are free, have few to no side effects, and can be started immediately.

SEEING YOURSELF AS AN ATHLETE IN TRAINING

When an athlete has a goal, he or she trains every day with that goal in mind. If you have the goal of a stable and happy life, free from the symptoms of bipolar disorder, you will also have to train every day in order to stay well. You must watch what you eat, what you do, whom you see, when you sleep, how much bright light you receive, and where you go. This is no different from what a top athlete must do in order to reach peak performance, and that's how you must look at your treatment plan: as a way for you to reach optimal brain health despite the bipolar disorder diagnosis. One goal of this chapter is to give you the tools to start this training process so that you can find the stability you need in order to get on with your life. These changes will take time, and you may resist them at first, but the more changes you make and the sooner you make them, the more chance you have of preventing another serious mood swing from taking over your life. Once again, as with any part of the treatment plan where you have to make choices, it's easier to create a plan and start these new behaviors when you're well, so that they are in place to help you when you get sick. If you're sick right now, baby steps are fine. It takes time to make some of these changes, so go easy on yourself.

■ *For Family and Friends*

All athletes need trainers. You can play a significant role in helping your loved one follow the ideas in this chapter. In fact, you can practice many of the tips right alongside him or her, offering your support and helping your loved one find stability instead of simply struggling while you watch.

Balia's Story

Age 50

Before I worked on my own response to my son's bipolar disorder, I felt like I was watching my son waste his life. He wouldn't take his medications regularly. He often stayed in his apartment with all the windows closed, even when it was sunny outside. I knew exercise would help, but he seemed to prefer to play video games and smoke cigarettes and pot. I never saw anything good in his fridge. I knew all about caretaking and knew that he had to be responsible for himself, but at the same time I knew that he had bipolar disorder and often *couldn't* take care of himself. He got very angry if I talked about the importance of light in the morning or suggested that we take a walk. I really wasn't sure what my choices were if he wouldn't listen to me and didn't seem to care about his health. So *I* changed. I simply came over and talked about bipolar disorder whenever he said things I knew were not him. I said, "That's bipolar disorder talking." I stopped blaming him for his bipolar disorder behavior. If he had cancer, I would be there for him. And I'm going to be there for him now. I put a small amount of food in his fridge and he ate it. I opened his windows and cleaned his apartment. It was for myself and not for him. I'm there for him and I feel better about my own behavior. These are very small steps, but we aren't fighting anymore. I know that as I make small changes in myself, I can help him get help as well—one thing at a time.

THE IMPORTANCE OF STRUCTURED SLEEP

One of the best ways for you to maintain stability is to keep a regular sleep schedule. Sleep is a powerful regulator of brain chemistry. A night of regular, uninterrupted sleep helps ensure that your hormones and neurotransmitters can do their jobs and give you the physical energy you need to get through the day. Of course, the difficulty is that sleep problems are one of the main symptoms of bipolar disorder, and it's often very hard to regulate your sleep when you're sick. The busy lifestyle many people lead today is another

■ *For Family and Friends*

If you're the parent of a young child with bipolar disorder, getting him or her on a very structured and calm sleep pattern can make an enormous difference in the management of this illness. Even if it's a struggle—and especially if mania is involved—do what you can to maintain a structure in the family and at least set an example your child can follow.

factor—regular sleep can be a luxury for people who work and have families. But research clearly shows that people with bipolar disorder must pay attention to their sleep and create a structured sleep schedule in order to stay stable. Upsetting your natural sleep patterns upsets the brain's ability to self-regulate, and can lead to mood swings.

Maintaining Structured Sleep

There are usually two types of sleep problems with bipolar disorder—sleeping too much and sleeping too little. One of the main challenges you face is to figure out if the sleep problems are caused by an outside factor affecting bipolar disorder, or if they come from the bipolar disorder itself. One thing is for sure: Sleep issues are *always* something you must take seriously and treat. There are three areas you need to watch in order to monitor your sleep:

1. Triggers: those environmental and stressful events that can disrupt sleep.
2. Medications, including over-the-counter products.
3. The illness itself.

Sleep-Problem Triggers

You always have to ask yourself: *Have I done anything to trigger these sleep problems?* Some triggers could include staying up too late a few nights in a row, social events, changing work or school hours, taking a trip to a new time zone, caffeine consumption, change in your diet to more stimulating foods, relationship problems, a large life change such as a new baby, or an upsetting world event. As you can see, there are many outside influences that can cause sleep problems. It can be quite frustrating when you just want to live a normal life and sleep when you wish—and yet the illness doesn't like serious sleep changes. Sleep disruption or deprivation is one of the most common triggers of mania, and even if you don't feel tired, missing sleep will interfere with the brain's natural processes for regulating itself. The goal is for you to recognize what factors disrupt your sleep and to eliminate as many as possible. The next chapter will cover triggers in detail, but for now, list your potential sleep-problem triggers here:

———————————————————————————————————

———————————————————————————————————

———————————————————————————————————

———————————————————————————————————

———————————————————————————————————

Medications

Bipolar disorder medications usually help stabilize and normalize sleep, but they also can produce sleep-related side effects (such as excessive sleeping or insomnia). You will have to watch yourself carefully so that you can learn what may be causing sleep problems: the disorder itself or your medications. If you're sleeping excessively since starting a medication, this is something you should talk to your doctor about. You will need to discuss dosage or possibly a medication change. Sleeping so much that you can't function is no way to live, and if this is the case, you will have to advocate strongly for yourself so that you can get the right medication at the right dose. On the other hand, some medications can inadvertently cause anxiety, edginess, and mania. If you're suddenly full of nervous energy and can't sleep after being depressed for a while, examine your medications and see if the side effects include restlessness and sleep problems. If so, you need to talk with your doctor immediately, especially if you feel manic. Over-the-counter medications, particularly decongestants and those used for weight loss, also frequently cause sleep problems. It's very important to keep your treating physician posted on any and all over-the-counter drugs you may be taking.

The Illness Itself

Depression and mania are notorious sleep disrupters. If you're already in a mood swing, it can be hard to tell the chicken from the egg. Depression can cause sleep disruption in three ways. The first is hypersomnia, or sleeping too much. Hypersomnia paradoxically often leads to extreme daytime fatigue. The second problem is insomnia. There are two common varieties of insomnia seen in depression: middle insomnia (tossing and turning and waking up numerous times during the night) and early-morning awakening (waking several hours before you want to get up and being unable to fall back to sleep). The third problem is a reduction in the amount of time spent in deep sleep, often due to caffeine, alcohol, and tranquilizers such as Xanax, Valium, Klonopin, Ativan, and others. Deprived of adequate deep sleep, people tend to feel very fatigued during the day and often start consuming more caffeine or using more tranquilizers or alcohol to sleep, when these are the very substances that can cause the sleep disturbance in the first place.

Anxiety is also a very common experience for those suffering from bipolar disorder. It often causes difficulty in falling to sleep—something professionals refer to as initial insomnia.

Mania affects sleep in an opposite way. Mania and hypomania are always accompanied by a markedly decreased need for sleep, *but without fatigue the following day.* If you begin to notice that you're starting to sleep a few hours less than normal at night (four or five hours a night, for example) and still feel full of energy when you wake up, this is a serious sign that mania may be starting, and you need to talk with your doctor immediately. Even though it probably feels great and you love having the energy, these good feelings rarely last, and the lack of sleep can lead to serious mood swings with often devastating consequences.

No matter what depression or mania does to your sleep patterns, you have to fight the desire to change your sleep schedule. Make a pact with yourself and pick a set bedtime. When you're depressed, tell yourself you can only get in bed and sleep at those times. During the day, avoid naps and do whatever it takes to make yourself get out of bed in the morning. Mania sleep problems are much harder to treat because they feel positive at first. So much gets done, and it's great not to be depressed. But this is a false sense of security. All manias need to be reported to your doctor and treated with medications even when you think it's just the real you coming out after a depression.

Fill in the following list to remind yourself what it feels like when mania starts to disrupt your sleep:

_____

_____

_____

_____

_____

ALCOHOL, TRANQUILIZERS, MARIJUANA, AND CAFFEINE ARE *NOT* TREATMENTS FOR SLEEP PROBLEMS

One thing is for sure: Alcohol, tranquilizers, marijuana, and caffeine are not solutions for sleep issues. They may seem like a solution, but they only add to and prolong the problem. It's very tempting to use such substances to regulate your sleep (or, in the case of caffeine, to combat daytime fatigue). They seem to work, which is why so many people self-medicate with these substances, but the truth is that they don't work in the long run. They're a mask for the symptoms rather than a solution, and you may find yourself with an addiction problem that truly exacerbates your mood swings. The reason that these substances are so dangerous is that their outward effects are quite different from what they actually do to your brain. Alcohol and tranquilizers, if taken in large enough amounts, can promote drowsiness and make it easier to fall asleep. However, it has been well documented that these drugs reduce the amount of time people spend in deep sleep and also often make depression a lot worse. Caffeine ingested in amounts above 250 mg per day can also reduce time spent in deep sleep. (This is explained in more detail later in the chapter.)

As hard as it is, try to limit these substances and look to more realistic treatments for your sleep issues. You can use accepted herbs such as chamomile for relaxation and peppermint for energy as well as homeopathic treatments or exercise for sleep issues. These solutions rarely have side effects and are less likely to cause you problems in the future. It's true that they don't seem to work as well at first, but over time your body can start to self-regulate; you will find you don't feel the need for the unhealthy substances as much as you used to. You really do have to think long into the future when it comes to what you put in your body. Don't add to your brain's regulatory problems by taking substances that affect your sleep and only make things worse.

The following are some helpful tips for avoiding sleep problems:

- Avoid working odd hours, especially shift work.
- Limit travel in different time zones.
- Set a go-to-sleep time and wake-up time, and stay in bed the entire time whether you're asleep or not.
- Create a sleep ritual that helps you get to sleep normally.
- Learn about natural sleep aids. (Always keep your physician posted about any and all over-the-counter and natural products you are using.)

■ *For Family and Friends*

If you party with a friend who has bipolar disorder, especially if he or she is manic, you are contributing to the illness. It may be that you met your friend in a manic phase, when he or she was the life of the party, and you probably miss that. But if you want to help your friend find stability, the partying has to stop.

■ Know what triggers your sleep problems.
■ Call your doctor at the first signs of mania.

This can be a daunting process if your work includes many of the issues addressed by the above tips. It really is up to you to decide if your lifestyle causes more problems than the job is worth. The journal section of this book (appendix C) includes an area where you can chart the number of hours you sleep. This can help you look for signs of mania and depression as well as keep your doctor informed of your sleep issues.

WHY YOU CRAVE JUNK FOOD

As you know, because you have bipolar disorder, your brain has trouble regulating itself. It's natural that you may want to treat bipolar disorder mood swings by eating foods that quickly increase energy and seem to lift your mood. The problem is that these quick fixes are often brought on by blood sugar changes, and are not an effective way to treat the mood swings. "Regular fluctuations in mood and energy are often linked to highs and lows in blood-sugar levels. These in turn are linked to the food we eat and drink, particularly sweet, sugary, and starchy foods. Such foods may temporarily fulfill a craving brought on by sudden tiredness and irritability, but they also cause our blood-sugar levels—and with them, our energy and mood—to seesaw. That's why, says Natalie Savona in *The Kitchen Shrink,* "Maintaining even blood-sugar levels is, therefore, one of the most crucial factors in improving our moods." It's actually more effective to *balance* moods with foods than to use food as a quick way out of a mood swing.

The Technical Facts About Food and Moods

There are three neurotransmitters that are especially important in mood regulation: dopamine, norepinephrine, and serotonin. These neurotransmitters are built from the essential amino acids tryptophan and tyrosine. The body doesn't naturally make tryptophan or tyrosine, which means they have to come from the foods you eat. Additionally, these amino acids enter the brain in small amounts. It has been found that certain dietary practices can increase the availability of the amino acids in the brain and at times have a positive impact on mood. Some suggestions include eating pure protein without carbohydrates, which will increase energy and combat fatigue; and eating complex carbohydrates with no protein to open cellular gateways. This allows more tryptophan to enter brain tissue, increasing serotonin levels, which can result in a reduction of anxiety.[1] The more you understand the way that food affects your brain, the better choices you can make when you eat. It makes sense that if you can use food and supplements to regulate your neurotransmitters, you may need lower doses of medications, which can mean fewer side effects.

THE BIPOLAR-FRIENDLY DIET

What you eat and drink affects your brain. You can see this if you eat a huge meal and then lose all your energy and feel like crawling into bed, or if you drink too much coffee and can't sleep. Bipolar disorder *is* affected by what you put in your body, and the more you can regulate the effect that food and drink have on your mood, the more you can manage your mood swings successfully. This is especially important if you live in an area that has less bright light in the winter, where it's normal to want to boost your mood with caffeine and sugary or white-flour-based foods that enter the bloodstream quickly and then potentially cause a mood drop as the effect wears off.

Omega-3 Fatty Acids

Omega-3 fatty acids are derived from diet, make up about 30 to 35 percent of brain mass, and are essential in making cell structures and carrying out intracellular biochemical reactions. These fatty acids are derived from fish and shellfish, and are also available in the form of fish oil capsules in your local health food store. Research strongly suggests that omega-3 supplementation (generally 2000 mg per day) along with medications can help stabilize mood in bipolar disorder.

What to Avoid

Foods made from refined white flour and white sugar may taste good, but they enter your bloodstream quickly, causing a spike in blood sugar and then a drop. This can adversely affect your moods. Try to add more natural sweeteners to your diet as well as whole-grain products. They really can make a difference in your blood sugar levels and promote stability. They can also be quite tasty. Yes, they are more boring than junk food, but this is a choice you have to make. Is it worth it to eat less junk in return for better moods? It's up to you.

Bipolar-Friendly Foods

The following are some bipolar-friendly foods that you can add to your diet:

- Whole grains for balance and fiber, such as brown rice or heavy whole wheat bread.
- Fruit for fiber and vitamins. This is a much better choice than candy or soft drinks.
- Tofu for the phytoestrogens that help regulate moods. Soft tofu has little taste and can be added to many foods.
- Dark green vegetables for vitamins and energy.
- Meat and eggs in the morning for protein.

Weight Gain

Weight gain is one of the main reasons people stop taking their medications. It's hard enough to be sick. When you add the weight gain on top of the mood swings, your situation may feel unbearable. There are some solutions to the weight gain problem. These solutions can help with weight gain due to medications, as well as that often associated with depression. It may help to once again think of yourself as an athlete in training. Athletes often have very restricted diets in order to reach their performance goals, and it may be that you will have to do the same in order to stay stable and physically healthy.

The following are signs that your medications are affecting your hunger:

- Feeling a bottomless pit of hunger.
- Feeling hungry even though you just ate.
- Eating if you wake up at night.
- Finding it impossible to stop eating—in fact, you eat without thinking about it at all, as though you are an eating machine.
- Gaining weight though your eating stays the same.
- Thinking of food obsessively—everything looks good.
- Feeling out of control with the constant desire to eat.

The best approach to medication weight gain is to reduce your eating and increase your exercise before you even have a chance to gain weight. This isn't fun and it's not fair, but if you want to find stability and keep yourself healthy, it's crucial. Considering that one of the main problems with many bipolar disorder drugs is an increased appetite, you absolutely must monitor your eating if your medications are giving you these troubles. If the weight gain starts quickly and seems out of your control, talk to your doctor immediately and ask for help. If you have already gained more weight than you find acceptable, there are a few steps you can take:

- Ask for help from a health care professional.
- Talk with your doctor about microdosing.
- Talk with your doctor about the newer drugs that have fewer weight gain side effects.
- Increase your exercise.

A Note About Hunger

It is almost impossible to describe the hunger caused by many bipolar disorder drugs. It is virtually insatiable—just as thirst can be insatiable with lithium. There are few things you can do about it. Weight gain is often inevitable, even when you eat less and exercise more. This is because some medications appear to change metabolic rates—how fast your body burns calories. Reducing caloric intake helps, but for some people it's often not a very successful option, especially with antipsychotic drugs and mood stabilizers such as Tegretol and Depakote. It is not abnormal for someone to gain fifty pounds on these drugs. Then there are some who do not gain weight at all and simply stop eating. It is a very complicated issue. The important thing is to not blame yourself. If you struggle with hunger and/or weight gain, be sure to mention it to your doctor. Some medication changes can help this problem. One of the main goals for drug developers is to create drugs with limited weight gain side effects, such as the antipsychotic Abilify.

- Reduce portions.
- Reduce the amount of fat, white sugar, and white flour in your diet.
- Increase the whole grains in your diet in order to control your blood sugar and increase metabolism.
- Join a weight loss group and get help from others in the same position.
- Work with a nutritionist who understands the challenges you face due to bipolar disorder medications.
- Prevent weight gain by making these changes now if you're newly diagnosed and just starting medications.
- Try some of the new medications that may help reduce weight gain, such as Topamax.
- Recognize that the hunger is drug-induced, and learn to live with it.

Don't Give Up

It may be hard to read the above list without making excuses for why you can't make the suggested changes. The number one solution for weight gain issues is prevention. If you're

■ *For Family and Friends*

If you have any responsibility for what a person with bipolar disorder eats and drinks (if you have a young child, for instance, or cook for a family member or partner), you can really have an influence in helping your loved one stay more stable and maintain a normal weight. The key things to remember are protein during the day and carbohydrates at night. This helps blood sugar remain stable. All athletes in training need a coach, and this is a role you can play if you know the facts about how food can regulate moods. Don't sit back and watch someone gain a lot of weight. If you see this happening, get help for your loved one immediately.

newly diagnosed and have just started medications, weigh yourself now and make sure to watch your weight carefully. People really *can* gain more than fifty pounds on some of these medications in a very short time. You don't want this to happen to you.

Caffeine

Caffeine is very seductive because it seems to help people regulate energy levels. It really does give you energy when you're tired, but it's a drug-induced energy. This means that

How Alcohol Affects Your Moods

Alcohol affects bipolar disorder in two ways: It causes depression, and it interferes with sleep. The problem is that it may seem to temporarily alleviate some depressive symptoms and help you fall asleep. This is the paradox that causes many people to use alcohol to self-medicate. The facts are that alcohol undermines sleep by significantly reducing the time spent in slow-wave sleep (more popularly known as deep sleep), and this affects the moods adversely by making you more depressed. Alcohol is not a treatment for mood swings; in the long run, it always makes bipolar disorder worse. Avoiding alcohol all together is your best defense.

Caffeine Consumption Questionnaire

	Average number of ounces/doses/tablets per day	Total mg per day
Beverages		
Coffee (6 oz.) 125 mg	_____	_____
Decaf coffee (6 oz.) 5 mg	_____	_____
Black tea (6 oz.) 50 mg	_____	_____
Green tea (6 oz.) 30 mg	_____	_____
Hot cocoa (6 oz.) 15 mg	_____	_____
Caffeinated soft drinks (12 oz.) 40–60 mg	_____	_____
Candy		
Chocolate candy bar 20 mg	_____	_____
Over-the-counter medications		
Anacin 32 mg	_____	_____
Appetite control pills 100–200 mg	_____	_____
Dristan 16 mg	_____	_____
Excedrin 65 mg	_____	_____
Extra Strength Excedrin 100 mg	_____	_____
Midol 132 mg	_____	_____
No-Doz 100 mg	_____	_____
Triaminicin 30 mg	_____	_____
Vanquish 33 mg	_____	_____
Vivarin 200 mg	_____	_____
Prescription medications		
Cafergot 100 mg	_____	_____
Fiorinal 40 mg	_____	_____
Darvon Compound 32 mg	_____	_____
Total mg caffeine per day		_____

Add up your total number of milligrams per day. Do you take in more than 250? If so, you should strongly consider ways to reduce this amount.

you need to keep having the caffeine in order to feel energized. It then builds up in your system and can destabilize your mood by affecting your sleep patterns. Caffeine is not a treatment for bipolar disorder mood swings. It only adds to the problems, especially if you have trouble with anxiety. Try to limit your caffeine consumption to 250 mg or less per day, and only have it in the morning (to avoid interference with sleep). Fill in the caffeine-consumption chart on the previous page to get a clear picture of how much caffeine you consume in a day, and then decide what is realistic for you. If you're consuming more than 750 mg of caffeine per day, it's a good idea to reduce your caffeine intake by 25 percent for the first week, and continue this rate of reduction each week until you reach a lower level (somewhere between 0 and 250 mg per day and, preferably, only in the morning). Even 250 mg (two cups of coffee) a day can interfere with sleep. This gradual reduction will allow you to avoid caffeine withdrawal. Many people find this easier to do by gradually switching from caffeinated to decaffeinated tea, coffee, or soft drinks. Many things about bipolar disorder seem out of control, but what you put in your body is totally in your control, especially concerning caffeine. Monitoring and regulating your caffeine intake is one of the cheapest and quickest ways to help yourself get stable, and it can really make a difference in your level of anxiety.

Why You May Get Sick More Often if You're Depressed

About 50 percent of depressive episodes cause a hormonal condition called hypercortisolemia, in which cortisol levels are extremely high. Cortisol is a steroid hormone that, at high levels, can cause potentially serious health problems. A sustained high level of cortisol can damage arteries and is being recognized as a risk factor in the development of heart disease. It also can contribute to increased risk of osteoporosis. Finally, when hypercortisolemia occurs for longer than six weeks, it can have a negative impact on the immune system. Cells of the immune system have been shown to function less effectively under such conditions. The result can be a less robust response to infections, and if a person so affected contracts a cold, the flu, or more serious infections such as pneumonia, the body may have a harder time fighting back. Recent studies indicate that bipolar disorder medications may be a defense against hypercortisolemia—which is another reason to make sure you find the right medications and stay on them.

BIPOLAR DISORDER AND EXERCISE

Why does exercise help to balance your moods? Throughout 99 percent of human history, all people had to be moderately physically active for at least two hours a day, just to survive as hunter-gatherers. It is built into our biology that movement is a normal daily experience, and it has been solidly demonstrated that exercise has a significant impact on the regulation of brain chemistry. Exercise and physical movement, especially repetitive movement, have been associated with stimulation of the production and release of the neurotransmitter serotonin. Elevations in serotonin have been found to have beneficial effects for some people experiencing clinical depression.[2] When you don't feel like exercising, try to remind yourself that you will feel a lot better afterward because the movement can change your brain chemistry and help you find stability. Regular exercise has also been demonstrated to be very effective in improving the quality of sleep. Just one hint: It's important to avoid exercising during the last three hours before retiring to bed. The immediate effect of exercise is to actually increase some stress hormones that may interfere with falling asleep, but these hormones are eliminated from the body after three or more hours and thereafter may help promote relaxation and sleep.

Taking a Walk

Walking can affect the mood-stabilizing chemicals you need in order to stay balanced. Exercise increases oxygen to your body, which can also affect your brain in a beneficial way.

■ *For Family and Friends*

Here's one way you can really make a difference. When you see depression start, it's especially helpful to go for a walk with the person, especially when it's light outside. Don't take no for an answer. Do it in stages. Don't ask how your loved one is feeling; just ask him or her to go for a walk with you because you want to walk: "I can see that you're depressed. I wish I could get rid of this depression for you, but I can't. I *can* help you get out and take a walk. This would mean a lot to me because it will help me feel I am making a difference in your life."

Exercise can also improve your immune system by suppressing the cortisol that often increases when you're depressed. There are just so many ways that walking benefits your moods. It really is the best overall exercise when you're feeling unmotivated and lethargic. Even a ten-minute brisk walk can result in more energy and often a noticeable shift in mood.

How to Start an Exercise Plan

If you're not a big fan of exercise, or if it seems impossible, then walking is a great first step. Just start to walk to your favorite music or to a book on tape, and with every step you take, remind yourself that you're changing your brain chemistry for the better. Picture the serotonin in your brain getting regular. Picture your moods getting more stable. Think of swinging your arms, looking at the sky, exercising your eyes, and using your mind to change your brain, and you may be amazed at how just ten to twenty minutes of walking every day can change your health. Start slow and make walking a part of your training. Walk with a friend to make it more enjoyable. Even better, take a hike and see something interesting. Once you see the benefits of walking, you may want to move to an aerobics class, yoga, tennis, or a team sport. The benefits of exercising with others are enormous: You get both the physical and the social contact you need to keep your brain healthy.

LIGHT

Why does light exposure affect bipolar disorder? Once again, for most of human history people lived outdoors and were exposed to bright sunlight each day. The human brain evolved in ways that were responsive to and dependent on certain environmental stimuli. Like exercise, bright light exposure has an impact on regulating certain neurochemicals that affect mood. The critical factor is the daily exposure to very bright light entering the eye and striking the retina. This activates a nerve pathway, the retinal-hypothalamic nerve, which goes to the hypothalamus, a brain structure that significantly influences mood states, sleep cycles, appetite, and sex drive. Because of this, natural bright light exposure is a critical factor in bipolar disorder mood swings. However, there needs to be a balance: For many people with bipolar disorder, too much light exposure can provoke mania, and too little can lead to depression. This is why hospitalizations for mania peak in the summer, and for depression, in the late fall or winter. There are strong connections

---

Light Exposure and Mania

Though commercially available light boxes can benefit people with depression during the darker months, it's important to know that people with rapid cycling or a tendency toward mania must always undertake bright light therapy under medical supervision, because light exposure is known to cause mania.

---

between seasonal changes in light exposure and bipolar disorder episodes. The key to successful treatment is to keep the amount of light exposure steady year-round. If you suspect that you need help regulating your exposure to bright light, talk to your doctor.

Starting Your Day Off Right

The way you start your morning can make a big difference in your moods for the rest of the day. Start the day with a plan for health. It may be very hard to get out of bed at first if you're depressed, or it may be hard to focus if you're agitated or slightly manic, but do it as often as you can and you will start to see results. Ask for help with this new plan and see it as part of your training for the future. The following list gives you a few ideas on how you can incorporate the suggestions in this chapter into your daily routine:

- Take a twenty-minute walk right after you wake up—ten minutes in one direction and then ten minutes to return home—to stimulate endorphins and serotonin. Make sure to pump your arms.
- Take 1000 mg twice a day of omega-3 fish oil. Keep your physician informed of this and all other over-the-counter preparations.
- Take a multi–B vitamin, and individual B vitamins such as folic acid and vitamin B_6, to help support the clearing of the stress hormones by the liver.
- Take supplements that support your immune system. Check with your doctor or naturopath on what will work the best for you.

Check the suggestions from this chapter that are realistic, everyday changes you are committed to making:

☐ Take a daily walk.
☐ Eat brown rice.
☐ Take fish oil supplements.
☐ Talk to health care professionals about bright light exposure.
☐ Exercise with others.
☐ Stop weight gain before it goes too far.
☐ Sleep at the same time every night.
☐ Talk about mania as soon as you have the first symptom.
☐ Cut back on caffeine.

MAKING THE CHANGES: WEIGHING THE BENEFITS AGAINST THE COSTS

There will be many times when you simply don't want to take care of yourself. You will want to goof off and eat junk and just ignore bipolar disorder. This is normal, but if it goes on for too long, it won't help you find stability. There will also be times when you will feel too ill to make the changes you want to make. Try to do what you can, and think of how much better you'll feel the next day, and the next. Think of the cost of not making changes and then think of the benefits of getting some bright light, taking a walk, watching what you eat, and sleeping regular hours. These benefits can be enormous, even with small daily changes. Once again, if you can remind yourself that you're similar to an athlete in training, it may make the changes easier.

SMALL STEPS THAT GET YOU WHERE YOU WANT TO GO

If you feel too sick today to make these significant changes, then make just one. Practice one idea in this chapter until you're ready to take on more. Bipolar disorder can wear you out. It can take all of your energy and often make you feel as though it has taken your soul as well, but if you treat the bipolar disorder first and don't take the symptoms personally, you can get better at practicing the ideas in this chapter. Do what you can now. In fact, just reading this chapter is a big step. Make one change today. And make another change tomorrow, and soon you can start to feel better. Small steps really do get you where you

Michael's Story

Age 33

When I was diagnosed with bipolar disorder, the doctors didn't really explain what would happen to my body. The medications seemed to make it change overnight. I used to be quite thin. Then I noticed that my stomach started to get a little round and that everything looked soft. I was hungry all the time. I didn't feel like exercising because I was so tired and sometimes all I wanted to do was watch TV and eat. I actually used to play some football and suddenly all I could do was zone out and watch it on TV. I knew I had to do something but after being in the hospital and then getting the news that I had bipolar disorder and that I would have to take medications, I just lost my energy for everything.

I went from being a pretty active person to one who sat around all day. I know my girlfriend was very upset with me. She was always saying, "Hey, let's go do this or let's go do that," and I just didn't have the energy. I could tell the medications were helping slightly. At least I wasn't getting manic. But at that point, mania felt better than this lethargy. Lying on the couch all day was enough to make anybody depressed. One day I just knew I'd had enough. I remember sitting up and thinking, *I have to make some changes or I will end up killing myself.* I was still pretty sick at the time and certainly didn't want to do anything I'd regret. I knew I had to do something to save my life.

So, I started by not letting myself stay in bed. I outlawed the couch. Period. No couch and no TV. As soon as I got up in the morning, no matter how I felt or what my brain was telling me, I went outside and walked for thirty minutes. I used to exercise a lot when I was manic before my hospital stay and so this seemed a bit like small time, but it was all I could do as the drugs made my bones feel like rubber. I did it every morning whether it was raining or sunny or cold. And I have to admit I started to see a difference. I know that it helped that I was getting light in the mornings again. I did this for a while and then decided to work on my diet. I went back to my natural way of eating and basically told myself I couldn't eat sugar all day. It's odd but before medications and before my diagnosis, sugar wasn't that important to me. But while I was on the couch I think I lived on chocolate junk food. So I did the walking, stopped the sugar, and have to admit I stopped smoking a certain something that for years I thought was a great treatment for mania. This took time and I went back to my old ways quite a few times. Then I realized I was needing less and less antianxiety medication. The voices I heard chattering in my head were getting better. I wondered if it was possible that the new life changes were making my meds work better? My doctor and I talked about lowering my medications. I went off my antipsychotics as the mania seemed kept under control by a mood stabilizer. I did all this on my own. People could offer me help, but it was ultimately up to me. I know that I'm the one that stood up one day and said, *I'm not letting this illness kill me. I'm taking charge of my own life,* and that's what I did. It's a lot of work. I have to watch for mania, but the depression has definitely lessened. I'm back to work and not on the couch anymore.

want to go. Forget the time it takes, focus on what you *can* do, and just do it every day, step by baby step; your future will show you the results. Scientific research has strongly demonstrated that consistent sleep patterns, diet changes, exercise, and appropriate bright light exposure at constant levels year-round can make a significant difference in maintaining stability, and are critically important for helping people get the best outcome in treatment for bipolar disorder. This is truly an area where you can make a great difference in your own moods without insurance, appointments, or extra money. Do what you can today to help yourself feel better tomorrow. The more you can work on these ideas and incorporate them into your life, the closer you can be to stability.

COMPLEMENTARY LIFESTYLE TREATMENTS FOR BIPOLAR DISORDER

There are further complementary lifestyle changes you can make to more effectively manage bipolar disorder.

- *Naturopathic medicine.* A naturopathic doctor is an excellent complement to your medications doctor because naturopaths are often educated in diet, herbs, body work, and other alternative treatments. Naturopathic doctors are also a good resource for learning new lifestyle-management skills that promote stability.

- *Homeopathic treatments.* Widely used in Europe to treat many illnesses, homeopathic medicines can help you with a variety of bipolar disorder symptoms, from sleep problems, anxiety, and physical issues to balancing the body and dealing with stress. Working with a licensed homeopathic health care provider can be an effective addition to your treatment plan. Please note that it is always wise to have health care professionals communicate with one another, especially when medications and any nonprescription remedies are being used, to avoid the possibility of drug interactions.

- *Body work.* Yoga, meditation, Reiki, chiropractics, acupuncture, breathing exercises, and therapeutic massage are some examples of the body-work options you can explore. It's not hard to see that your body can be out of balance when your mind is out of balance. It makes sense that treating the balance of the body can help the mind, as well. There are many treatments and paths you can explore in this area. A gentle yoga class (including pranayama—yoga breathing) from an experienced and intuitive teacher can make a world of difference, as can acupuncture, shiatsu, or chiropractic treatment. You may also want to try:

  Chi gong and tai chi.
  Dance therapy.
  Art therapy.
  Working with animals.
  Energy healers.
  Macrobiotic diet for depression, and other nutritional approaches.

BIPOLAR DISORDER AND CHANGE

Lifestyle management for bipolar disorder always includes regulating the different areas of your life. This can be a very difficult process at first. Bipolar disorder may have controlled your behavior for a long time, and it's hard to know what you need to regulate to find stability. *One easy way to approach lifestyle management is to simply acknowledge that your bipolar disorder brain doesn't like a lot of change.* Of course, bipolar disorder often makes you crave change, which is why the lifestyle changes step of your treatment plan must include an effective and easy-to-follow action plan so that you can override what bipolar disorder wants and focus on what *you* want and need.

For most people without bipolar disorder, superbusy or unstructured lifestyles do not lead to major mood swings. Most people *can* stay up all night doing a project or traveling on a plane, then get some sleep the next day, without causing any problems. You probably can't. Your brain simply can't regulate the chemicals that are needed to keep you stable through these changes. Many people can drink coffee, alcohol, go to a party, have a few stimulating discussions, and get up and go to work the next day. You will probably get sick from this behavior, especially if you do it regularly. These are just the facts, supported by well-controlled research studies,[3] and the sooner you accept them and make the lifestyle changes you need to make, the sooner you can find stability. Upcoming chapters will give you many specific suggestions to help you with these changes.

Your Toolbox

Knowledge about bipolar disorder.

A correct diagnosis.

A list of your major symptoms.

Medication knowledge.

Help with side effects.

A regular sleep schedule.

A bipolar-friendly diet.

A daily walk.

Regular, appropriate bright light exposure.

CHAPTER 3

WORK AND MONEY

Bipolar disorder is notorious for causing work and financial problems. From depression to mania and everything in between, the illness can seriously impair your ability to work effectively and manage your money. These work and money problems can also affect you in other areas, including your ability to get health insurance and the quality of relationships with the people in your life, especially those who may judge you because you can't work the way they think you should. Many people with bipolar disorder simply can't handle the stresses of everyday work. Bipolar disorder is an illness that is often triggered by outside events, and for many people, work is one of the biggest triggers.

Work and money problems can also affect your self-esteem and your hope for the future. You may wonder what the future holds for you if you have trouble working and currently can't make enough money to support yourself. You may have made some big financial mistakes when you were sick that now cause significant stress in your life and impair your ability to get better and move on. The good news is that there are solutions to these problems. It takes time, but a comprehensive treatment plan can often help you find enough stability so that you can work effectively and make the money you need to support yourself in the future.

This chapter helps you get a realistic picture of your current work and financial situation, so you can decide what kind of work you can do while still maintaining your stability. It also helps you get a current financial picture, offers tips on how to get help if you are in a financial crisis, and covers disability and where you can go for information on what to do when you are unable to work and support yourself.

For Family and Friends

This may be the hardest chapter for you to read. It's often the family members who feel the burden of a relative who can't work or make much money. Friends are often affected by this as well. Our society ties so much self-worth to career and financial stability, so it's natural that the behavior of people with an illness that causes work and financial problems would create misunderstandings and frustration all around. Many people with bipolar disorder struggle with this constantly. The more you can understand why your loved one may not be able to work or make money right now, the more you can help him or her get better and create a plan that can allow for going back to work in the future.

THINKING ABOUT WORK AND MONEY

When you're sick, this may be a topic that you wish would just go away. It's hard enough to deal with treating this illness, especially if you were recently diagnosed or spent time in the hospital. Thinking of work and money may seem overwhelming right now. This chapter will gently guide you through the process so that you will at least have a clear picture of where you stand, and help you ask for the assistance you need.

FRIENDS AND FAMILY MEMBERS

Do your friends and family members question you about your work ability and the trouble you have with money? It's possible that people are frustrated with your lack of current work, and may not understand that it's often a part of the illness, and not always something you can control. It might help to read this chapter with your friends and family and ask for their help with the exercises. It may be that they can be more understanding when they see that work and money issues are a problem for most people with bipolar disorder, and that you're not alone if you struggle with finding your place in a world that emphasizes work and making money.

SHAME, EMBARRASSMENT, AND WORRY
ABOUT WORK AND MONEY

You may have a lot of painful emotions surrounding your work and financial situation. Our society places a high value on working and making money, and if bipolar disorder has affected your ability to work and earn, you can easily feel like a failure. For many people, not being able to work the way they know they're intellectually capable of working is one of the most devastating side effects of this illness. You may feel worthless and ashamed at your inability to do what is expected of you, especially if you have a family you can't support or have to ask for financial support from family members and friends. It's also terribly hard to come out of a severe manic or depressive episode and face the work and financial mistakes you made while you were sick. Some people go home from the hospital to thousands of dollars of debt, having lost everything they worked to build. Does it help to know that you're not alone if this has happened to you? Shame, embarrassment, and worry over work and finances are a large part of having bipolar disorder for many people, and the sooner you can accept that this is just another part of the illness that needs to be treated and prevented, the sooner you can make some positive changes to make sure it never happens again. You're not the exception if your work and financial life are a mess. You're certainly not without hope.

THE PRESENT

The first step to getting your work and financial position back on track is to see where you are with work and money right now. The clearer you are on how you feel and where you

■ *For Family and Friends*

There is a good chance that your loved one has caused some family financial problems. Sometimes you just have to accept the consequences of this illness and then do everything possible to help make sure the big problems are prevented in the future. And yes, this may include limiting contact with someone who refuses treatment and continues to make disastrous financial decisions.

Robert's Story

Age 39

My sister never really did any real work as far as I was concerned. She was just sort of a perpetual student. She worked at a few jobs but seemed to leave them early. If she had a way not to stay at the job, she would just leave. She moved a lot. It's as though she didn't care. She was never in a state of mind to keep a job for a long period of time. Personal issues at her jobs were too much for her. Then she was diagnosed and started a treatment plan. She made a *lot* of changes. Now when she has an idea that will make money she's able to do it. She still gets sick and depressed and sometimes she is way too talkative and goes out too much and does things that make her more ill, but nothing like before. She just has to take it easy. It takes her longer, as she gets sick when she takes on too much, but she's pretty amazing.

want to be in the future, the better able you will be to make decisions on what you need to do now to improve your situation.

How You Feel About Work

A person's ability to work is often taken for granted. It's simply what a person does. When you have an illness that takes away this ability to work, you can have some serious internal conflict about who you are as a person and what your future will be like. Answer the following questions regarding work to get a clear idea of how you feel about your current work situation.

How does bipolar disorder affect your work abilities?

_____

_____

_____

_____

_____

How does work affect your bipolar disorder symptoms?

_____

_____

_____

_____

_____

What changes would you like to make regarding work?

_____

_____

_____

_____

_____

What are your work goals for the future?

_____

_____

_____

_____

_____

How You Feel About Money

Depending on how much you have been able to work in the past, your financial situation may be quite serious as well. Once again, it may help you to know that you're not alone if you have significant financial problems because of this illness. Answer the following questions regarding money to get a clear idea of how you feel about your current financial situation.

How does your bipolar disorder affect your moneymaking abilities?

_____

_____

_____

_____

_____

How do your financial problems affect your bipolar disorder symptoms?

_____

_____

_____

_____

_____

What changes would you like to make regarding money?

_____

_____

_____

_____

What are your goals for the future regarding money?

_____

_____

_____

_____

Orlanda's Story

Age 25

It's tough being diagnosed with bipolar disorder. My whole life changed. My dreams for who I wanted to be just seemed to disappear. I cried a lot when I realized that all the years of searching for the "right work"—in other words, work I could handle without getting fired or leaving due to stress—was really about an illness and not about my ability to move forward in life. I know my family looked at me like a failure. I felt like a failure. I was supposed to be successful just like all of the people in my family. My father is a professor. My brother is a lawyer and my mom is a principal of a middle school! Everyone, including me, had ideas of where I should be. I just couldn't get there. I felt like someone or something had stolen my life from me. Work is just so important. I had a friend from France once tell me I worried about work too much. "Work is just something you do for money," he said. "Real life is about friends and family." I wanted to believe him, but I wasn't even able to work for money! I had to go on disability for almost a year after my suicide attempt. I honestly thought I would never work again. And if I did get better, what work could I possibly do? I realized that the high expectations I had for myself would have to change. I would have to look for something that fit into the diagnosis, as I knew for sure that a busy, stressful job would make me even more ill. Time has helped a lot. I manage this illness every single day. I'm not one of those people who takes a pill and goes back to the high-pressure job. I had to make changes. I now work as a graphic designer for a small firm instead of a large one. It's less money and certainly less glamorous, but I can stay well. Everyone knows about the bipolar disorder. I've taught them how to help me stay stable. No, this is not the work life I expected for myself. I had to change my expectations. I am so proud of myself now! Five years in the same job and no more visits to the hospital. I am a success.

Now that you're more aware of how you feel regarding your current situation, you're ready to get a clear picture of your past experiences with work and money. You will then use all this information to create a plan for your future.

For Family and Friends

Family members and friends can definitely help with the work and financial history sections of this chapter. Think back as far as high school in order to get a clear picture of your loved one's work and financial history. People with bipolar disorder who were diagnosed later in life usually have a checkered work history, and seeing it all on paper can be stressful. Still, it's a needed tool to help your loved one get realistic about what he or she can do now instead of blaming him- or herself for the past.

CREATING A WORK HISTORY CHART

It's important that you look at your past work history in order to get a realistic picture of your future work prospects. It may be that medications will work well for you and that you will be able to work normally. If this is not currently the case, however, it's important that you be realistic about what you can and can't do at this time regarding work. If you just came out of the hospital, it may take some time before you can go back to work, and you may have to take on unexpected jobs until you are well enough to return to your regular work. The following exercise will help give you a complete picture of your work history; you can use the information to decide what work you can do realistically in the present and near future.

Chronological work history. List as many jobs as you can remember with dates and an explanation of why you left:

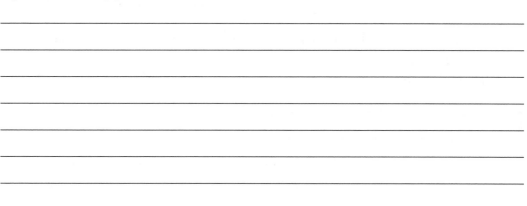

Patterns. What patterns do you see when you look at your work history?

_____

_____

_____

_____

_____

Money. How much money did you make each year in the last ten years?

_____

_____

_____

_____

_____

Current work situation. What is your current work situation? If you're working, how many hours do you work? What is the pay? Are you staying stable?

_____

_____

_____

_____

_____

Future prospects. Considering your past experiences and your bipolar disorder diagnosis, answer the following questions:

What is likely to be your work ability in the next six months?

_____

_____

_____

In the next year?

_____

_____

_____

In the next five years?

_____

_____

_____

What is different in your life now that will make your work prospects more positive in the future? Some answers could include medications and this book:

_____

_____

_____

Now that you have a realistic picture of your past and current work situation, you can create a plan for the future. The tips in this book, along with the right medications, can make a huge difference in your life, and you may find that your future work prospects will be better. Or maybe you have always had trouble with work in the past and will continue to have trouble in the future if you don't make changes now. The above exercise will at least give you an idea of where you are in the moment and what steps you need to take next. The following section will help you do the same with your financial situation.

CREATING A FINANCIAL HISTORY CHART

The next step, after looking at your work situation, is to look at your financial situation in a realistic way. It makes sense that where there are work problems, there will be money problems. You can use the following exercise to help you get a clear picture of where you are financially.

Getting a realistic picture of your finances can be very distressing, especially if you just got out of a bad mood swing. But considering how sensitive bipolar disorder is to stress, the worry brought about from *not* knowing where you are financially can be worse than facing the reality of your situation. Writing down exactly where you are financially gets it out in the open and can take away some of the fear of the unknown you may feel. No matter how worried you are about filling out the next chart, try to do it anyway. Then you will know exactly where you need help.

Your Debts	*Your Assets*
Housing: _____	Cash: _____
Car: _____	Savings: _____
Credit cards: _____	Investments: _____
Loans: _____	Housing: _____
Medical bills: _____	Car: _____
Miscellaneous: _____	Miscellaneous: _____
_____	_____
Total debt: _____	Total assets: _____

A realistic picture of the future. Look over the yearly salaries you listed in the work exercise, and then look at your present situation. What can you realistically expect to make in the next month, six months, and year?

One month: _____

Six months: _____

One year: _____

Can you survive on this money? _____

Steps you need to take to support yourself in the future: _____

_____

_____

_____

Knowing your financial history and your current financial situation can take away some of the fear associated with how this illness will affect your future. You can say to yourself, *I'm in debt and I can't work right now because of bipolar disorder—what do I need to do next?* Or maybe you will find that your situation is better than you thought. The good news is that using the tips in this book can make a major difference in your work and financial futures. The following section will offer some suggestions on how to get back on your feet and prevent future work and money problems.

RECOVERING FROM AND PREVENTING MANIC DISASTERS

No matter what has happened in the past because of bipolar disorder, you always have the ability to make things better in the future. The future may not look exactly as you expected it to, but you can recover from the disasters caused by the choices you made when you were manic. If you had a severe manic episode that created financial ruin for yourself and/or your family, then welcome to the bipolar disorder club. You're not alone! Maybe your disaster happened on a small scale, or maybe you're now in bankruptcy because of the episode. This happens to many people with the illness. Your goal is to set up checks and balances so that you never again have to go through a financial disaster because of bipolar disorder. The following list is a good beginning:

- Take your medications. This is the only way to truly prevent serious manic episodes.
- Create the habit of writing down everything you spend and showing it to someone daily if needed.
- If credit cards are the problem, then you will have to get rid of them or let others hold them for you. Debit cards and checkbooks can be a problem as well. Going to a cash-only system is a good step, even if it's embarrassing.
- If you're in a relationship or live with someone you trust, create a weekly check-in where you go over all of your financial decisions and determine if you're getting manic. There is a space for you to determine your current mood in the journal at the end of this book. This can't stop just because you start to feel more stable.
- Have a regular health care appointment (even if you feel well) in which you can be monitored for mania.

- If you're married, you may want to have all financial accounts in your partner's name, including any retirement and investment accounts, so that you don't have access to these accounts when you're ill. Once again, this hurts, but you may have to do it.
- Accept that mania is going to affect your life financially, and that one way to protect yourself from this is to prevent the mania by using the tips in this book as well as those from your health care professionals.

Answer the following questions to get started on your own checks-and-balances plan:

What checks and balances can you start today?
Who can you ask for help?
Do you have credit cards? Is it realistic for you to use them?

■ *For Family and Friends*

Manic spending is a loaded topic. Many family members and friends often either don't notice or ignore the subtle signs that mania is starting, then grow very upset when the damage reaches thousands of dollars. If you have anything to do with the finances of someone with bipolar disorder, you must protect yourself first. This means working together as a family (or as a friend) to see the early signs of mania. You may need to make the decision to help and support your loved one emotionally, but *not* financially, unless he or she is monitoring the mania.

DEPRESSION, WORK, AND MONEY

For many people, depression is the main source of work and money issues. Getting things done when you're depressed often feels impossible—and work is obviously about getting things done. There are tips in this book on how to prevent depression from reaching this stage. As with mania, prevention is the best way to make sure that depression does not affect your work.

For Family and Friends

How do you feel when you see your loved one sit on the couch or stay in bed all day? You probably want to yell and say, "What are you doing with your life? You need to get up and face the world and take care of yourself! I can't be responsible for you." To be honest, this won't work—depressed people often simply can't respond the way you want them to. The illness is too strong. Depressed people sit around all day without working because this is a part of bipolar disorder. The only thing that will work is treating the depression. This book has a variety of tips for ending depression and getting back to life. This is the first step to getting back to work.

HOW TO DISCUSS BIPOLAR DISORDER AT WORK

Bringing up bipolar disorder at work can feel impossible for many people. There is still a large stigma attached to mental illness, and being honest about bipolar disorder may be difficult at first. It may be that your past behavior was bizarre and difficult to explain; if you have tried to kill yourself, the topic may feel too overwhelming to broach. It's up to you to decide how much you want to reveal to your co-workers and management, but in many cases you may find that being honest and asking for help can release some of the burden and fear you feel surrounding this illness. Many people know about bipolar disorder these days due to the attention it has received in the media. There are many tips in this book on how to talk to people about the illness, as well as ideas on how you can involve helpful people in your treatment plan. You will have to decide what you need to do re-

Your Legal Rights at Work

Your legal rights at work regarding taking time off and other issues will depend on where you live. Talk with your human resource or personnel department about your situation. You can also talk with a local mental health organization and your doctor regarding your rights.

garding your work. Keeping your illness a secret may be more stressful than telling the truth and asking for help. Ultimately it's up to you to assess the response you might get at work and make your decision accordingly.

DISABILITY

There may come a time that you're simply too ill to work and support yourself. If this happens, you may have to look into disability to help yourself financially until you're stable enough to go back to work. Though many people who go on disability remain on it, having a goal of using it temporarily until you're more stable and more able to support yourself is a much more positive approach. Never forget that bipolar disorder, when treated comprehensively, can and often does get better. Disability requirements are different depending on where you live. Talk with your doctor about your eligibility. Remember that the process can seem overwhelming at first, but it's worth it if you need time off work to treat the illness so that you can get back on your feet. Disability does not have to be forever. It really can be an interim decision you make until you are ready to return to the work world. It's nothing to be ashamed of.

What Is Disability?

In the United States, the term *disability* refers to the assistance provided by the Social Security Administration. This assistance is broken into two categories: Supplemental Security Income (SSI) and Social Security Disability (SSD). SSI eligibility is determined by a person's income, while SSD eligibility is determined by whether a person is able to work for the next twelve months. When a person goes to the Social Security department to apply for disability, he or she actually applies for SSI and SSD on two separate forms, but is potentially eligible for both forms of assistance.

There are two appointments involved in applying for SSI or SSD. The first requires you to go to the office to officially apply for disability. The second involves an in-depth evaluation of your case. Applying for disability can be quite daunting. The following section can help you with the process.

■ *For Family and Friends*

Disability is not failure. If your loved one had cancer and could not work, you would not consider it a failure. Bipolar disorder, too, is a serious illness, and needing time off from work to get better is normal. This is especially true after a hospital stay.

Finding an Advocate

If you're ill and unable to work, there is a good chance that the disability application procedure will be quite stressful. One way to help yourself through the process is to find an advocate to go to the appointments with you. This can be a family member, a friend, a social worker, or someone who has successfully been through the process already. If your life is in chaos because you're sick, can't work, and have money problems, then it's very important that you ask for help from someone who is calm, organized, and able to help you through the process.

Here are some tips that can help you when applying for disability:

- When asked why you're at the SSI office, have a reply ready such as, "I have a bipolar disorder diagnosis and am unable to work. I would like to apply for assistance."
- At the first meeting, find out exactly what paperwork you will need for the next session. Make a list of this paperwork.
- Be ready for more paperwork than you want to deal with. Use a specific folder for all papers you receive, and keep this with you. (See chapter 9.)
- Take someone with you to the appointments. The wait can be long and quite stressful if you're already sick.
- Know what will happen before you get there by researching the process on the Internet.
- Utilize the services of NAMI (National Alliance for the Mentally Ill), DBSA (Depression and Bipolar Support Alliance), and DRADA (Depression and Related Affective Disorders Association).

- Have a list of questions you want to ask when you get to the counter.
- Try not to go to the offices on a Monday or a Friday—these are the busiest days. Midweek mornings are best.
- Create a bulleted list of your health history that mentions dates of hospital stays and any other important information. Use the charts in appendix C for help.
- If you were in the hospital, make sure you have a copy of your admitting evaluation and discharge diagnosis paperwork to put in your file.
- If you don't have a social worker, find someone who knows the social service system and can help you get through the application process.
- Be very aware of the amount of money you will receive, and don't be confused by the fact that it may come from two places—SSI and SSD. This does not mean you are paid twice, but that the total amount you receive will be split between the two departments.
- Once the office has your paperwork, they will ask for official records from the state regarding your illness. Your complete file will then go to a determination committee, which can take six months or more to make a decision. This means that you will have to find a way to get financial help while you wait for the determination.
- If your application is rejected, it's a good idea to immediately file an appeal. It's not abnormal for someone to be denied the first time, especially in the case of a dual diagnosis. You may want to hire a lawyer who practices disability law to help you with your appeal. Such lawyers often get paid only if your appeal is successful.

■ *For Family and Friends*

If you're able to help your loved one apply for disability and go through the process smoothly, it's a gift he or she will always remember.

Knowing the System in Your Area

It's important that you know how the system works in your area. In the United States, your county health system is the main resource for information on what is available. If you're already in this system, you will be assigned a caseworker to help you with the disability application. The county can help you find information on low-cost therapy and help with the cost of medications. You can also use the Internet resources listed in appendix A to help you find information on what to do if you don't qualify for disability and don't have insurance. Many of the mental health advocacy groups such as NAMI, DBSA, and DRADA offer information on how and where to find help. Appendix A has a list of their contact information.

Knowing That Disability Doesn't Have to Be Forever

Disability is something you can use to help yourself financially while you're working on your new treatment plan. You can use it as a time to help yourself become stable enough to go back to regular work. Needing disability to help you get back on your feet is nothing to be ashamed of.

ALTERNATIVE WORK OPTIONS

It may be that the work you envisioned for yourself is not possible because of bipolar disorder. You may have to find work alternatives in order to support yourself and maintain your stability. This can be depressing in itself, but it may have to happen in order for you to stay well. High-powered jobs with a lot of obligations or deadlines may be a trigger for your symptoms, as can working with stressful people. A job that enables you to work in a nonstressful environment may be the best way for you to maintain stability. Looking for alternatives does not have to be a demeaning or sad situation. When you look at your work and money situation realistically, you can make a simple one-year goal regarding work that will ensure that you have the time to create your 4-Step Treatment Plan, get your medications stabilized, and work on your relationships. You can then make different work choices when you are more stable.

SCHOOL

School problems tend to mimic work problems, and this makes sense when you realize that it's the people interaction, obligations, and deadlines that often make work a difficult place for people with bipolar disorder. School has all of these demands and can be just as stressful for people as work. Many people with untreated bipolar disorder have a checkered school history, especially those who have a tendency to pull all-nighters to study for exams. If school is currently your issue, you can use the ideas in this chapter to help you get a clear picture of your ability to go to school in the present, and to see what might be possible in the future. You can also look into the Americans with Disabilities Act to see if you qualify for special assistance.

SLEEP PROBLEMS DUE TO WORK AND SCHOOL OBLIGATIONS

As you read in chapter 2, a significant cause of bipolar disorder symptoms is work or school schedules that affect sleep. Shift work is a main source of symptoms, as is exam time in school. It is imperative that your sleep schedule remain stable if you want to successfully treat this illness. This may mean changing jobs or taking fewer classes at school.

DEALING WITH A WORK OR FINANCIAL CRISIS

Whether you have just come out of the hospital, maxed out your credit cards while manic, or made detrimental bipolar disorder decisions regarding work and money when you were depressed, there are solutions to these problems. They may take awhile and they may be daunting at first, but you *can* make it out of some terrible situations if you have a plan for stability and then a plan to take care of your current work and financial situation. The following are some tips for getting through a crisis situation:

- Ask for help from the right people.
- Ask for a letter from your doctor explaining the illness, which you can then send to your creditors.
- Call your creditors and consolidate your debt. Talk honestly: "I have an illness called bipolar disorder. One of the symptoms of this illness is excessive spending

when I'm manic. I just went through a manic episode where I made some very poor financial decisions. I have a letter from my doctor explaining this situation. I would like to know what I can do to arrange paying off this debt."

- Go to consumer credit counseling—but only if there is no fee and the organization is legitimate.
- If necessary, explain your situation honestly to the people where you work.
- Keep your doctor's appointments.
- Stick to your treatment plan in order to prevent the mood swings from going this far again.
- Take your medications faithfully.
- Remind yourself that it's money and that you're alive. It may take years, but you *can* turn around your money situation.

Now that you're starting a treatment plan for bipolar disorder and learning to manage the illness comprehensively, there is a good chance that you can improve your work and money situation greatly. You can learn what it is about work that triggers your symptoms and find work that better fits your lifestyle. You can learn to prevent the mood swings that cause financial problems and ask for help for any problems that you have now due to the illness.

■ *For Family and Friends*

Even after reading this chapter, you may still feel completely frustrated and out of control in the situation with your loved one. It's surely the case that you did not expect to have to support someone too sick to work. But as you've read in this chapter, work and money problems are completely normal when someone has bipolar disorder. And unfortunately, you may have to be the one who supports your loved one until he or she is able to go back to work. Or maybe it was your money that got spent during a manic episode. The ideas in this chapter can at least help you set up your own checks and balances to protect yourself in the future. If you can work together with your loved one to prevent serious mood swings, this is the best defense against work and money problems due to bipolar disorder.

This chapter has been a quick overview of a very serious topic. Work and money issues are so bound to bipolar disorder that they may seem impossible to mend. As you probably know, lifestyle changes due to work and money issues can be significant at first. But the situation can and often does get better. Give yourself time to fill out the exercises in this chapter, and then make some small decisions that will take you where you want to go in your future. If you have had years of untreated bipolar disorder, you may have a lot of work and money messes to clean up, but you can do it. It just takes time and planning.

Your Toolbox

Knowledge about bipolar disorder.

A correct diagnosis.

A list of your major symptoms.

Medication knowledge.

Help with side effects.

A regular sleep schedule.

A bipolar-friendly diet.

A daily walk.

Regular and appropriate bright light exposure.

A clear picture of your work history.

A clear picture of your current financial position.

BEHAVIORAL CHANGES

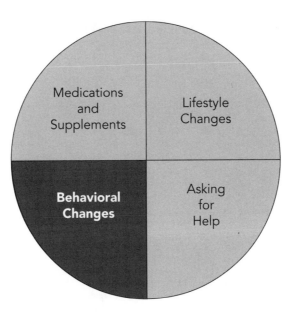

CHAPTER 4

KNOWING YOUR BIPOLAR DISORDER TRIGGERS

The next step of the Take Charge 4-Step Treatment Plan teaches you to recognize, examine, and ultimately change the behaviors in your life that adversely affect bipolar disorder mood swings. You could literally spend the rest of your life treating bipolar disorder symptoms with medications and various lifestyle changes, but if you continue to repeat the behaviors that trigger the symptoms in the first place, you may stay in constant crisis-control mode instead of learning to manage the illness effectively. Medications, supplements, diet, and exercise are all excellent tools for managing the illness, but without an understanding and management of your triggers, stability may remain elusive.

It's often hard to know why you get sick in certain situations. You may feel like the world is a difficult place for you and that you're oversensitive to normal life. This happens because for many people, bipolar disorder symptoms are triggered by outside events. This chapter will help you examine your personal triggers and what you can do to recognize and modify them, and then will offer you tools to prevent them from making you ill. Trigger control is about prevention and can take away a lot of the stress you feel when

Why Prevention?

- Prevention is more effective than constant crisis control.
- Prevention is often free.
- It saves trips to the doctor and hospital.
- Preventing bipolar disorder symptoms helps relationships stay stable.

> ■ *For Family and Friends*
>
> The importance of family members and friends regarding trigger manage-
> ment cannot be stressed enough. There are so many areas where you do
> have control over what a person with bipolar disorder experiences. As you
> read this chapter, think about and take notes on how you contribute to bipo-
> lar disorder triggers and what you can do in the future to minimize their im-
> pact on your loved one.

faced with managing your illness. Next to medications, this can be your most powerful
management tool. If you have insurance problems or money issues, trigger management
is one of the most cost-effective ways to treat bipolar disorder.

IDENTIFY YOUR TRIGGERS TO HELP
PREVENT BIPOLAR DISORDER SYMPTOMS

When you experience stress—both good and bad stress—it activates a number of nervous
system and hormonal responses. The stress hormone cortisol is released from the adrenal
gland, and the neurotransmitter CRF (corticotropin-releasing factor) is released in the brain.
These normally help mobilize an adaptive fight-or-flight response. In mood disorders,
however, too many of these molecules are released, and one main effect is that excessive
CRF and cortisol begin to significantly interfere with sleep—especially by obliterating
deep sleep. Sleep disruption or deprivation is a well-known trigger for mania and hypomania. Also, both excessive CRF and cortisol can directly cause changes in the brain that
lead to depression. For people with bipolar disorder, these changes are known to also disrupt internal mechanisms (called second messengers) in certain nerve cells (such as norepinephrine), resulting in a loss of their ability to self-regulate. Mood swings are the result.

In other words, when a normal brain is faced with stress, the nervous and hormonal
systems react as they should. The person feels stress and his or her brain, operating like an
effective shock absorber, can respond and then quickly return to homeostasis. The result
is some stress symptoms but no major mood swings. When the bipolar disorder brain is

faced with stress, on the other hand, it reacts abnormally. Stress symptoms arise, but the brain fails to regulate emotions and more severe mood symptoms can erupt. If you can learn to recognize and ultimately prevent your main bipolar disorder stressors (triggers), then you can bypass this incorrect response and create more stability. It makes sense that if you don't give your brain the chance to react with a mood swing, you have a better chance of managing the illness.

FACING REALITY IS HARD

It would be nice if people with bipolar disorder could just all take a pill and never experience bipolar disorder symptoms again. Though a few people with the illness do experience amazing symptom relief from medications, the majority still struggle even when the medications are working. Because of this, most people with bipolar disorder must carefully monitor their triggers in order to stay stable even when they are taking medications. In general, the medications help the random mood swings and help people with bipolar disorder stay more stable in everyday life, but as soon as a big trigger happens—a car wreck, a wedding, the death of a loved one, the birth of a baby—they can go right into mood swings again. Medications can definitely make the mood swings less serious and, in many cases, less lengthy, but the swings are still triggered if you aren't careful and very aware of your triggers.

WHY YOU GET SICK WHEN GOOD THINGS HAPPEN

Many people associate stress with bad situations. But the truth is that stress can occur from good situations as well. As you know, your brain has trouble regulating itself when presented with change. Just because you want the change, such as starting a new job or graduating from school, doesn't mean your brain can tell the difference. For your brain, change is often a trigger for bipolar disorder. People can become manic and psychotic when they're marrying the person they love. They can go into a deep depression after the birth of a much-wanted child. Bipolar disorder does not differentiate between whether you want the change or not. It only sees change and reacts.

As you learned in the first chapters, your brain is different from normal brains. It reacts differently. Bipolar disorder is often a stress-induced illness, which means that any

■ *For Family and Friends*

It may be hard for you to understand how on earth a person with bipolar disorder can get sick when something good happens—a new relationship, graduation, the birth of a child, or a promotion at work—but this is because you don't have bipolar disorder. Your brain probably works normally. It has appropriate reactions to events. The bipolar disorder brain has inappropriate reactions. When you experience a happy event, your brain usually responds with happiness. The stressed bipolar disorder brain often sees the happy event as a stressor that is no different from a negative event. Even if the person with the illness truly is happy and wants to respond to the event with happiness, his or her brain will not let this happen. Desire for a good outcome is no defense against bipolar disorder. The best approach is prevention. You will see that the journal section of this book has a place to list possibly stressful situations well before they happen. You can help your loved one prepare for these events by walking through them before they happen. What mood swing might show up because of the events? What thoughts can be expected? What behaviors? Does your loved one need more medications? You can also make sure that a doctor's appointment is set up during the time of the event for a bipolar disorder checkup. No, this is not overkill. This is how you help your loved one prevent hospital visits and possible disasters caused by serious mood swings. An outsider such as yourself is often able to see problems before they happen, while the person with bipolar disorder is often too caught up in the positive situation to notice the warning signs of illness. It's easy for you to feel rejected when the person with bipolar disorder gets sick on such a special occasion—especially when the event is very positive and important to you. Prevention is the key to making sure your event is not ruined and that you and your loved one can enjoy it.

change that can cause stress—whether good or bad—has the potential to make you ill. You simply respond to stress differently than most people. A marriage may be wonderful and something you have looked forward to, but as the day gets closer, your brain feels the stress that the wedding is causing in your body and responds with mood swings. A new

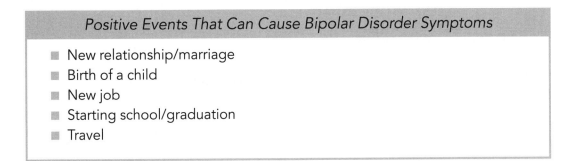

> ### *Positive Events That Can Cause Bipolar Disorder Symptoms*
>
> - New relationship/marriage
> - Birth of a child
> - New job
> - Starting school/graduation
> - Travel

baby, a new job, or a big trip can be exciting and wonderful in many ways, but for you, they may cause serious mood swings that make you doubt your true feelings and can wreck many relationships. You can become manic and psychotic during final exams even though you're well prepared and ready to graduate. You can become suicidal from the news that you have won an award or that you finally landed a new work contract that means your business will double. When you accept that all major change has the potential to trigger bipolar disorder, then you can learn to treat the illness by recognizing and modifying potential and known triggers instead of wondering what is wrong with you.

What Triggers Bipolar Disorder?

The following list shows some common bipolar disorder triggers. This list can be a bit overwhelming at first, as it seems that life in general triggers bipolar disorder. It may not be possible to avoid all of these triggers, but just knowing that they can cause mood swings is the first step in preventing problems. The more of these that you can modify and eliminate, the more chance you have for stability. As you read the following list, put a check in the box next to the triggers you already know cause you problems so that you can be ready for them in the future.

- ☐ Drug and alcohol use/abuse.
- ☐ Sleep disruption/deprivation/erratic sleep patterns.
- ☐ Shift work.
- ☐ Relationship problems—especially with difficult people involving arguments or abuse.
- ☐ Travel.
- ☐ Work/school.

☐ Chaotic lifestyle.

☐ Poor diet with no exercise.

☐ Caffeine.

☐ Medications, including antidepressants, steroids, and stimulants.

☐ Change of any kind.

☐ Move to a new location.

☐ Anything new, such as a new baby, new relationship, new job, or new school.

☐ Obligations and deadlines.

☐ Taking on too much.

☐ Lack of a set schedule.

☐ Opiate drugs such as Vicodin.

☐ Over-the-counter products such as SAM-e, St.-John's-wort, and weight loss products (like ephedra).

☐ Enjoyable social events.

Doesn't it sometimes feel like you have to monitor *everything* in order to stay stable? It can be frustrating and sad to realize that this illness can be triggered by so many outside influences. But just as those with diabetes need to monitor their diet and insulin levels, you will have to monitor the triggers of bipolar disorder in order to maintain stability. As you find more stability, there is a good chance that you will not react as strongly to triggers and may be able to tolerate a lot more change in your life.

Discovering Your Personal Triggers

Knowing your personal triggers is a strong tool to add to your treatment plan. Once you determine what triggers cause each of your major bipolar disorder symptoms, you can work on modifying and hopefully eliminating them. This is a very inexpensive way to prevent the

---

Medication Triggers

Medications can trigger bipolar disorder mood swings. Talk with your doctor about medication side effects if you have started a new drug and are suddenly experiencing rapid cycling, mania symptoms, or suicidal thoughts.

mood swings. One result of managing triggers may be that with better control over mood swings, at some point you may be able to be treated with lower doses of medications (thus reducing medication side effects). Trigger management can also result in improved relationships, and the ability to work and support yourself in the way you want to live. Discovering your personal triggers may take some time, but the results can be significant.

The following exercise will help you discover these triggers so that you can create a plan for modifying and preventing them in the future. Trigger examples are listed under

---

Alex's Story

Age 50

I used to obsess about everything that was wrong with my life. How could someone have so many problems? I just couldn't get happy. I was always bored or sad or dysfunctional. I tried therapy and read so many books, and yet I still had these problems. It was like having a low-grade flu all the time. I couldn't figure out what I was doing wrong. Then everything changed. I read about triggers and how they affect bipolar disorder symptoms and I had the thought, *What if these are bipolar disorder emotions that are triggered by outside events and I really don't have a ton of problems? What if I worked on the triggers instead of focusing on what I felt like all the time?* I noticed that the weather, certain people, stress, work, and life in general could trigger these feelings of being unhappy and dissatisfied, even when I was okay the day before. So I started working on the triggers. Now I know what thoughts and feelings come up with certain triggers. When this happens I usually get caught up in the bipolar stuff and I start searching for what went wrong, and then I stop myself and say, *Wait a minute! This is a bipolar disorder feeling. Nothing is wrong. Nothing has changed. What triggered this?* And then I work on the trigger and try not to repeat it in the future. I still feel that low-grade emptiness once in a while, but I understand it better. There is nothing wrong with my life. There is something going on in my brain that triggers that thought. Working on triggers changed my life.

> ### ■ *For Family and Friends*
>
> Family members and friends are often much better trigger detectives than the person with the illness. Create your own list of the triggers you see and, if possible, compare lists with your loved one to create the most comprehensive trigger list possible.

each symptom. You can then write your own ideas on what triggers your personal symptoms and think of ways to modify and eliminate these triggers. (It may be helpful to ask a family member or friend to help you with this list.) The section lists examples of the symptoms you may experience. You can follow the same process with any symptoms not covered in this section.

YOUR TRIGGERS

Look over each symptom, read the examples, and add your own triggers.

Depression. Poor diet, lack of exercise, relationship issues, staying at home all day, lack of contact with people, meds that aren't helping, drinking at night, lack of purpose, feeling that there's nothing to get up for, _____

_____

_____

_____

_____

Mania/hypomania. Staying out late, being around stressful people, taking a business trip, family problems, lack of day-to-day structure, arguing with your partner, trying a light box, exposure to upsetting or stimulating media, very stressful job, planning a wedding, _____

_____

_____

_____

_____

Paranoia. Starting a new class with new people, depression, lack of medications for psychosis, doing too much, crowds, _____

_____

_____

_____

_____

Anxiety. Caffeine, taking on too much, starting a new project at work, having no time to exercise, forgetting to breathe deeply, _____

_____

_____

_____

_____

Irritation/anger/aggression. Depression, taking on too much, not getting enough sleep, an overstimulating new antidepressant, poor relationships, trouble at work, _____

_____

_____

_____

_____

Cognitive problems. Depression, medication side effects, taking on too many projects, trying to do too much, mania, overstimulation, _____

_____

_____

_____

_____

Obsessions/compulsions. Depression, psychosis, staying up too late, caffeine, starting a new relationship, anxiety, new job, _____

_____

_____

_____

Feeling overstimulated. Saying yes to everything, meeting new people, too many social events, going to the mall (or any other high-stimulus place), _____

_____

_____

_____

WHAT YOU CAN DO

Look over each symptom, read the suggestions, and then add your own ideas.

Depression. Change my diet, walk for twenty minutes each day even when I'm too tired, talk with my doctor about meds, do something I love every single day, ask for help, find something to look forward to, _____

_____

_____

_____

Mania/hypomania. Talk with my doctor and get meds that help, set a bedtime and stick to it, avoid caffeine, cancel some obligations, work on relationships, find some balance, turn off the television, recognize the desire to party or travel on a whim as a symptom that needs treatment,_____

_____

_____

_____

Paranoia. Remind myself this is a normal bipolar symptom, try not to act on the thoughts, talk to my doctor about psychosis, limit stimulation in new situations, _____

_____

_____

_____

Anxiety. Take a few days off from obligations, do yoga, do breathing exercises, walk, avoid caffeine, meditate, _____

_____

_____

_____

_____

Irritation/anger/aggression. Check my meds, stop caffeine, ask for help, treat the depression/mania first, refuse to act on my thoughts, _____

_____

_____

_____

Cognitive problems. Learn my medication side effects and ask my doctor for help, take on less so that I can concentrate better, work on the depression, work on mania, _____

_____

_____

_____

_____

Obsessions/compulsions. Do less until the obsessions stop, talk with my doctor about psychosis, work on anxiety, focus on treating the illness instead of focusing on a person, say no when my brain won't be quiet, set limits on computer and cell phone use, _____

_____

_____

_____

_____

Gray's Story

Age 42

My mother used to be really weird if she had a fight with someone and they yelled at her. It would automatically make her suicidal, and she told me she would hear a voice that said, "You would be better off dead." This was from an argument! That's all. It seemed ridiculous to me. Get over it! Really, why blow things out of proportion like that. I used to tell her to calm down a lot. She didn't like that too much. I had to be so careful around her and never get angry or say something with a loud voice. I didn't want to make her suicidal. And then she got diagnosed with bipolar disorder. When we heard about triggers and that suicidal thoughts were a common reaction to a trigger such as an argument, it made a lot more sense. She's such a smart lady, and all this emotional stuff just seemed so odd in someone who was so smart. Now she manages the illness in many ways, and one of them is to tell people she can't and won't argue with them. If they yell, she walks out of the room. And if the suicidal thought comes up she says to herself, *This is a normal reaction to a bipolar disorder thought. I do not have to listen and I certainly don't want to die.* I'm impressed with how vigilant she has become about taking care of herself. I always loved her. Now I admire her.

Feeling overstimulated. Stop everything extra for a week to calm down, say no even when it's hard, avoid crowds, _____

_____

_____

_____

_____

BEING PREPARED FOR THE BIG TRIGGERS

Sometimes, no matter how hard you try to stay stable, the big triggers of life can make you ill. The end of a relationship, a legal battle, getting fired, the death or illness of a loved one, and world events simply happen. Many people end up in the hospital after these triggers because they didn't have a plan in place to treat bipolar disorder first, the minute the trigger happened. You know that your brain is different and that even with the right medications, it may respond to stressful triggers with a mood swing. If you're ready for these triggers with a plan to notice the first signs that a mood swing is starting, you can imme-

■ *For Family and Friends*

If you are going to participate in a large event with a loved one such as a vacation or a family reunion, you have every right to make a list of your concerns and discuss them with your loved one. Here is an example:

- I know that sleep problems cause bipolar disorder symptoms. Do you have a plan for the time change while we are on vacation?
- In the past, you've become very overstimulated and angry at family events. What can we do together to make it different this time?

Though this may feel like babysitting, it's not. It prevents wrecked events and saves relationships.

diately call your doctor, read this book for ideas, ask your friends and family for help, and watch yourself closely. This can save money, time, and your relationships and prevent serious mood swings. Being prepared for the big triggers can prevent serious mood swings and save your life.

DUAL DIAGNOSES

A dual diagnosis occurs when a person with bipolar disorder also has a drug or alcohol addiction. As seen in the trigger lists in this chapter, drug and alcohol abuse will always cause bipolar disorder problems. The facts are very clear. If you abuse drugs or alcohol, the statistics are grim. It makes total sense that you may have turned to alcohol and drugs to self-medicate. This is a serious illness with very uncomfortable symptoms. Many people go for years without being diagnosed, and often create their own way of dealing with the illness. This often leads to the dual diagnosis. You may have used alcohol or drugs to help you manage the mood swings so that you can get on with your life. Unfortunately, there is no easy solution if you have a drug or alcohol problem, but there is hope. If a person with a dual diagnosis can find medications that regulate the brain chemistry, create a comprehensive treatment plan that works, and ask for help, there's a good chance that the moods can become more stable so that the alcohol and drug addictions can be treated effectively. If you're in this situation, get help for the drug and alcohol problems as you read this book by attending a substance abuse recovery program or a 12-step program, and constantly remind yourself that while you may have had some darn good reasons to use alcohol and drugs to self-medicate, you're now starting a treatment system that truly can make a difference. This may be unbelievably hard, but as your bipolar disorder symptoms lessen it's often the case that your use of alcohol and drugs may lessen as well. When you treat bipolar disorder effectively, your need for the alcohol and drugs can change. Use this knowledge to motivate yourself to get help.

HOW TO MANAGE AND PREVENT YOUR TRIGGERS

Though there are some triggers you can't avoid, many are in your control. The more aware you become of these triggers, the better your chances of finding stability. There is a section in the journal at the end of this book (appendix C) where you can monitor your triggers and plan ahead for any known event that might cause you problems. Once you create a plan for bipolar disorder triggers, you can have more control over the illness. It helps to know that you don't necessarily have to stop something completely; a break may be all you need. The following list will help you to manage and prevent your triggers:

- Know the first signs that you're getting sick. This includes the first things you say, do, and think when a mood swing is starting.
- Teach the people in your life what to look for to know you're sick so that they can help you.
- Identify the trigger of the symptoms by examining your life.
- Leave or modify the situation if necessary.
- Avoid the trigger in the future.

The better you know your personal triggers, the easier it will be for you to teach others what you need. If someone wants to argue with you, you can say, "I can't do this right now. I have to take care of myself or I'll have a mood swing." If someone wants you to go to an overstimulating social event, you now know that the consequences may be a mood swing. You can be honest with the person and ask for his or her understanding when you have to decline an invitation. Saying no to potential triggers is a powerful tool in treating this illness. Knowing, modifying, and ultimately stopping your bipolar disorder triggers are your strongest management tools, as they are the areas where you have the most control.

Trigger management is another free tool to add to your bipolar disorder treatment plan. It may take some time for you to become more aware of what causes your bipolar disorder symptoms, but once you have a list of the more common triggers, you can make the changes needed to stop them from making you sick. This can be difficult if the triggers are something you enjoy doing or if they are caused by friends or family members, but sometimes the hard decisions are the ones that help you to find the most stability. It's all about balance when it comes to triggers, and the more big triggers you can stop, the better you will be able to handle the little ones when they come along. The behavioral changes you start today may take some time getting used to, but once you see the results, you will not want to go back to living in chaos from day to day instead of truly managing your environment and your reaction to it.

■ *For Family and Friends*

Family and friends often trigger bipolar disorder symptoms in the person they love. Sometimes this is done inadvertently—the person with bipolar disorder can be so darn sensitive, you may feel like you have to tiptoe around so he or she won't get sick. This can be very tough on you, especially if you are a friend who just wants to have fun. There are probably many ways you help your loved one, but there are also some very obvious and quite serious ways you can make a person with bipolar disorder more ill. Here are some of the trigger behaviors you can look out for in yourself:

■ Arguing.
■ Getting really angry at the person for bipolar disorder behavior.
■ Pressuring the person about work or money.
■ Not understanding mood swings. Feeling as if the person is sick out of defiance—this is especially true for teenagers with bipolar disorder.
■ Telling the person who has just been in the hospital or who has gone through a really tough mood swing that he or she should "be better by now."
■ Punishing someone for obvious bipolar disorder behavior.
■ Considering a hospital visit a weakness.
■ Living a stressful life yourself that affects your loved one.
■ Creating a noisy, stressful living environment.
■ Goading the person to go out, drink, or live like before he or she was diagnosed. ("What's wrong with you? You used to be so much fun!")

It's terrifically frustrating and unfair that you have to watch your behavior simply because someone in your life is sick, but unfortunately it's the reality of having someone with bipolar disorder in your life. You must remind yourself that your loved one is seriously ill and that you play an important role in helping maintain the stability you both have worked so hard to establish.

Your Toolbox

Knowledge about bipolar disorder.

A correct diagnosis.

A list of your major symptoms.

Medication knowledge.

Help with side effects.

A regular sleep schedule.

A bipolar-friendly diet.

A daily walk.

Regular and appropriate bright light exposure.

A clear picture of your work history.

A clear picture of your current financial position.

A list of your bipolar disorder triggers.

Tips to modify and stop the triggers.

CHAPTER 5

THE BIPOLAR CONVERSATION

Have you ever noticed that bipolar disorder affects the way you communicate with the people in your life? It's normal to find holding a regular conversation with someone difficult if bipolar disorder is controlling what you think, say, and do. The people in your life can become frustrated, angry, confused, and just plain worn out from trying to decide whom they're talking to when you're sick. This communication problem is one of the main reasons you may have relationship issues in your life.

Now that you're more aware of your bipolar disorder symptoms and their triggers, you're ready to learn effective tools for preventing the common communication problems caused by bipolar disorder. This illness can be very sneaky. It can affect what you say, think, and do without your knowing that it's in control. Once you learn to recognize the language and actions you use when bipolar disorder is talking for you, you can stop the illness from taking over your life, ruining your relationships, and causing you to make decisions you don't want to make.

■ *For Family and Friends*

This is a critical chapter for family members and friends. When you learn to spot and prevent the bipolar conversation, you can literally end many of the communication problems caused by bipolar disorder. So many things about this illness are out of your control. This is one area where you can be in complete control and truly help your loved one manage and ultimately prevent serious mood swings.

This chapter teaches you to recognize and prevent the troublesome conversations caused by bipolar disorder that often upset your relationships. It gives you tips on how to teach the people in your life what to look for so that they can help you prevent these communication problems. The ultimate goal of the chapter is to teach you to recognize the language you use when you're sick, and to see it as a sign that you need help so that you can prevent bipolar conversations before they even get started.

THE BIPOLAR CONVERSATION

How can friends and family members possibly say the right thing when you tell them, "I'm a failure and I want to die"? How can they know how to respond to your anger, paranoia, or mania language? Most people react to this bipolar disorder language by taking it seriously and trying to talk you out of what you're saying. They react to your words literally, and this usually starts something called the bipolar conversation. Because bipolar disorder can take away your ability to reason, you often say and do things that are more about bipolar disorder than about anything you really think and feel. If you're unaware that bipolar disorder is doing the talking for you, the result can be a circular conversation where you keep talking like an ill person, and yet the person you're talking to reacts as though you're in a normal state but for some reason just can't see the facts. The problem is that this conversation seems very real for you *and* for the person you're talking to. This means that not only do you need to recognize the signs that a bipolar conversation is starting, but your friends, family, co-workers, and all the members of your health care team need to learn the signs as well. If you can both see that bipolar disorder is doing the talking, you can then treat the illness instead of having a pointless and frustrating conversation.

The following examples show the typical bipolar conversations that can result from depression, paranoia, anger, mania, and anxiety. Notice what the person who is having the mood swing says, and then look at how the person listening gets caught up in the bipolar conversation and interprets it very literally. Notice the language that the person with bipolar disorder uses, and how the listener reacts to it.

■ *Depression talking.* "I don't think I'll ever be happy. It just seems like my life is always like this. Nothing makes me happy. Nothing tastes good or feels good. I see no point in a life like this. I just can't live like this anymore. I'm tired of how everything goes wrong for me all the time."

Miranda's Story

Age 40

Here's how my partner talks when he's depressed: "Just leave me alone. Can't you see that I'm in one of those moods? Why do you want to bother with me anyway? I know you'd be better off with some other person who has an appetite and wants sex." I used to think—*Appetite? He eats. Sex? Well, we still have sex and it's good sex, unless he's in one of these moods. What in the world is he talking about?* And I would try to talk to him for hours and get out of him what was really wrong. Did he want to leave me? Was I doing something? And then a really strange thing happened. I heard about the bipolar conversation that Julie Fast wrote about in her first book. And I started to watch what he said when he was depressed. It was exactly what he'd said the time before when he was depressed, and the time before that! I couldn't believe it. We had been having the same pointless conversation for years. "I don't see why you stay with me." And my reply, "What's wrong? Don't you love me anymore?" And then things just seemed to pass and we would get back to normal. And then it would start again and I'd be like, "Oh no. Not this." Now I know what it is. It's depression talking and nothing more. I no longer let it go any farther than the first sentence. And what's great is that he usually catches it himself. He'll say a few things and then go, "Oh, God, I'm depressed again." And we know to get out the treatment plan we use for his depression and focus on that instead of focusing on a fake problem in our relationship.

Reaction. "Wait a minute. What do you mean you'll never be happy? You've got a new baby and lots of friends. If food doesn't taste good, maybe there's something wrong with you physically. You have so much to live for. I think your life is great. Why are you so sad? What's wrong? I don't understand why you feel so miserable when things are going so well. Can't you just accept your life and enjoy it?"

■ *Suicidal thoughts.* "I don't want to live anymore. My life is a mess and I no longer want to get out of bed in the morning. Things are just too hard and you'd be a lot better off without me. I think it's time for me to just take care of things and end this. I'm so tired of being such a failure and a burden." (Starts to cry.)

Reaction. "Oh, God. You're scaring me so much. We just got married! What are you talking about. Don't you love me? What about the things we talked about just a few weeks ago? The new house and the trip to Hawaii? Why have you changed like this? I love you so much. Please don't kill yourself. What would I do without you?"

■ *Paranoia talking.* "All my friends are too busy for me. I can tell I don't even matter to them. They have their own lives and I'm sitting here alone all the time. I feel so lonely and they don't even notice. I think they're tired of me and maybe have decided that I'm not worth the friendship. I get the feeling that they're talking about me to each other because I'm such a problem. I know that my boss looked at me really oddly at the staff meeting today."

Reaction. "What are you talking about? You have plenty of friends and you had lunch with one today. Why would they talk about you? This is a bit weird. You're not alone all the time. Why do you need so much attention? You need to let other people lead their lives and just get on with your own life. Wait! You told me just last week that your boss said you were doing a good job! What's wrong with you?"

■ *Anger talking.* "Just leave me the hell alone! Why are you crowding me and telling me what to do? Mind your own damn business and get out of my face. Why do you want to bother me all the time and ask me so many stupid questions? I just need some space!"

Reaction. "Don't you talk to me that way! What do you mean I'm crowding you? I'm just talking with you! Why are you so angry all the time? I'm tired of it. Everything sets you off. You need some anger management! I'm sick of this. Your moods are wrecking my life!"

■ *Mania talking.* "There's nothing wrong with me! I just feel good for once. Can't you just let me have some fun? Do you want me to stay depressed forever? I'm finally happy and all you want to do is ruin my fun."

Reaction. "I don't want to ruin your fun, but I don't understand you. Just last week you were tired all day, and now you're up all night writing and listening to music. I can't keep up with you. I just want to know what's going on. Why have you changed so much? I'm really worried that you'll burn out again. Can't you just slow down a bit?"

■ *For Family and Friends*

Do you see yourself in these bipolar conversations? It's such a normal human reaction to want to talk someone out of obviously unreasonable thoughts. And yet, as you probably know from experience, this does not work at all when someone is in a serious bipolar disorder mood swing. In the following section, your loved one will write down what he or she thinks they say in certain mood swings. You can do the same exercise and write down what you hear them say in certain mood swings. It will be interesting to compare what your loved one *feels* he or she says in the illness with what you *hear*.

■ *Anxiety talking.* "I have to get out of here. I can't breathe. I feel like the walls are pressing in on me. My chest hurts! I can feel pains in my ribs! I can't breathe!"

Reaction. "Oh, God! What's wrong? Are you sick? Do I need to call a doctor? What's wrong with you? This is scaring me. Do you need a paper bag? Is it a heart attack? I don't know what to do!"

As you can see, it's so easy for your friends and family members to get caught up in what the illness makes you say. The good news is that there is a solution. The best way to prevent these conversations is for you and all of the people in your life to recognize and write down the specific language you use during each major bipolar disorder symptom.

Your Bipolar Conversations

Write down what you say when you have the following symptoms:

Depression: _____

_____

_____

_____

_____

Suicidal thoughts: _____

_____

_____

_____

_____

Paranoia: _____

_____

_____

_____

_____

Anger: _____

_____

_____

_____

_____

Mania: _____

_____

_____

_____

_____

Anxiety: _____

_____

_____

_____

_____

Recognizing Your Leading Comment

When you look at your conversations during mood swings, you may realize that you repeat a particular sentence every time you get sick. This is called the leading comment—the first thing you say when you start a mood swing. For example, your first comment when you're depressed may be, "I don't have any friends." When you're manic, it may be, "I'm finally feeling good again and it's time to have some fun." If you're paranoid, you may say, "People are looking at me funny." These are leading comments that often cause terrible problems in the lives of people with bipolar disorder; they are the comments that start the bipolar conversation, and the person listening has no idea what's going on. Problems ensue. These leading comments upset the people in your life because they're not based on reality but are a symptom of bipolar disorder. If they go unrecognized, entire conversations happen that are in the control of bipolar disorder, and the relationship often experiences serious difficulties. As a result, you may find yourself without the support you need. Recognizing the leading comment is the first step to preventing the bipolar conversation from ruining your relationships.

The Leading Action

Sometimes the beginning of a bipolar conversation is not a comment but a physical action. Some leading actions include crying, sighing, shortness of breath, pinched lips, or any other physical sign that you're sick.

Under each of the major bipolar disorder symptoms listed on the pages that follow, read the examples and then write your leading comments and actions. These examples cover just a few of the major symptoms of bipolar disorder. You will need to learn the leading comments for your other major symptoms as well.

■ *For Family and Friends*

As a family member or friend, it may be that you clearly recognize the leading comment and action when your loved one is ill. There is also a good chance that he or she is totally unaware of this behavior. If this is the case, you can write down the leading comments and actions that you notice in your loved one and use this information to help you stop *your* part of the bipolar conversation. You will learn that you can't get involved with the leading comment and you must see it for what it is: a sign that the person is potentially ill and needs help. People with the illness may grow offended if you say, "Oh, this is the bipolar conversation, and I'm not going to talk to you right now." The point is to understand that a bipolar conversation is starting and use the tips in this chapter to keep it from going farther. Walking away when you see one starting does not help anyone. As with all of the tips in this book, you as a family member or friend may have to walk a fine line in order to help without seeming controlling, intrusive, or upsetting to the person with bipolar disorder. The role you have to play can be frustrating for you. Still, remember the alternative: arguments that escalate out of control because your loved one is ill. You can at least improve your level of stress and frustration by *responding* instead of *reacting* to the bipolar conversation.

Depression. "I never do anything right." Crying, sighing, slumped body language,

_____

_____

_____

Suicidal thoughts. "I don't want to live anymore." Crying, rolling in a ball, limp body, making no eye contact,_____

_____

_____

Paranoia. "My friends are calling everyone except me." Wearing a sad or confused look, becoming teary, _____

_____

_____

Anger. "Don't stand so close. Why do you always have to crowd me and get in my business?" Balling fists, pinching lips, narrowing eyes, _____

_____

_____

Mania/hypomania. "I just can't believe how good I finally feel!" Smiling, eyes very wide and clear, practicing good posture, _____

_____

_____

Anxiety. "I can't breathe." Feeling that the walls are closing in, being short of breath, wearing a panicked look,

_____

_____

How to Tell the Difference Between the Bipolar Conversation and the Normal Conversation

How do you know if something is a leading comment instead of a regular part of a conversation? There are two ways. First, leading comments stay the same every time you have the same symptoms. For example, depression leading comments will be the same every time you get depressed. You won't come up with something new each time. There is a definite pattern. Second, the comments are rarely true. They're manufactured by an ill brain. If you step back and analyze the comments, you can see that they're one-sided and represent all-or-nothing thinking. Once you learn the pattern of these comments, you can see they're a sign that you're sick and need to treat bipolar disorder first, instead of acting on the comments. One way to do this is to teach your friends and family members how to talk with you the minute they hear the leading comment or see the leading action.

> ### ■ *For Family and Friends*
>
> As a friend of someone with bipolar disorder, there is a good chance you have been on the other end of a paranoid bipolar conversation. These conversations are often started by e-mail or in a phone message. You will read or hear what your friend has to say and probably think, *What on earth is she talking about? I'm not upset with her, and I don't want to stop being friends! This is ridiculous. She needs to get some self-esteem and grow up!* This paranoid conversation often ends friendships. It's very important that you talk about this with your friend *before* it happens. Create a way that she can tell you what she's feeling, talking to you about the paranoia and getting your help instead of taking it out on you.

LEARNING TO RESPOND INSTEAD OF REACTING

The following section offers tips for how the people in your life can respond to you and help you when you're ill, instead of reacting to what you say. You can learn to do this with yourself as well. It's as though the "well you" can rationally respond to the "ill you" so that you can get the help you need. Most people have the same bipolar conversation every time they get sick, so once you learn your own patterns, the conversations will be easier to recognize and stop before they go too far. Sometimes you will be able to recognize your own bipolar conversations, but for the most part you'll need to rely on the people in your life.

Teaching Others Not to React to Your Bipolar Conversation

The following exercise can help the people in your life learn to recognize and respond to the bipolar conversation. The initial remarks are the same as the ones listed above, but notice how the listener has learned to spot that bipolar disorder is talking. The person recognizes the leading comment, and instead of getting into the pointless bipolar conversation,

> ■ *For Family and Friends*
>
> The day you learn to respond instead of reacting to the bipolar conversation is the day you know you're finally getting somewhere in your own experience of dealing with this illness in your life. You may feel you're in some kind of control when you tell your loved one what to do and think in order to get better; it can be hard to let go of this. Still, as tough as it is at first, there is a lot of relief when you finally get used to the technique and stop letting bipolar disorder control your conversations.

he or she focuses on the real problem: The person is sick and needs help with bipolar disorder.

■ *Depression talking.* "I don't think I'll ever be happy. It just seems like my life is always like this. Nothing makes me happy. Nothing tastes good or feels good. I see no point in a life like this. I can't live like this anymore. I'm tired of how everything goes wrong for me all the time."

Response. "This doesn't sound like you. This sounds like depression is talking. You sound depressed. I have some ideas on how to help you. Do you think your medications are too low? How about if we go take a walk and discuss what we can do to deal with this depression? I'm concerned that you might be having suicidal thoughts. I want to help you get through this depression." (Notice that this person doesn't ask, "How can I help you? What do you need?" A depressed person cannot respond normally to these questions. The solution is to take action yourself.)

■ *Suicidal thoughts.* "I don't want to live anymore. My life is a mess and I no longer want to get out of bed in the morning. Things are just too hard and you would be a lot better off without me. I think it's time for me to just take care of things and end this. I'm so tired of being such a failure and a burden." (Starts to cry.)

Reaction. "Oh, no. You're really sick and I'm taking you to the doctor right now. Did you change your medications? You told me that this happened before and you were better once you went to the hospital. I know this is bipolar disorder talking. We just got married and it was too much for you, wasn't it? We were worried this might happen, and now we're going to do something about it. I love you so much and I know you want to be with me, but for right now we have to go to the hospital and get this bipolar disorder under control."

■ *Paranoia talking.* "All my friends are too busy for me. I can tell that I don't even matter to them. They have their own lives and I'm sitting here alone all the time. I feel so lonely and they don't even notice. I think they're tired of me and maybe have decided that I'm not worth the friendship. I get the feeling that they're talking about me to each other because I'm such a problem. I know that my boss looked at me really oddly at the staff meeting today."

Response. "I've heard you talk like this before. I know it seems very real to you when you feel this way. Bipolar disorder is telling you these things again. I'm a friend and I don't consider you a problem, but I do think you need some help. Have you talked with your doctor? You taught me to notice the signs that you're paranoid, and I hear the language you always use when you're stressed and the paranoia starts. What can we do right now to take care of the bipolar disorder?"

■ *Anger talking.* "Just leave me the hell alone! Why are you crowding me and telling me what to do? Mind your own damn business and get out of my face. Why do you want to bother me all the time and ask me so many stupid questions? I just need some space!"

Response. "Wait! I know you don't want to talk to me this way and it's very hard for me to keep my temper when you do, but this sounds like bipolar disorder. Have you been having mood swings? I want to help you. I know you don't want to treat me this way. Let's work together and take care of this."

■ *Mania talking.* "There's nothing wrong with me! I just feel good for once. Can't you just let me have some fun? Do you want me to stay depressed forever? I'm finally happy and all you want to do is ruin my fun."

Response. "Oh, boy. This sounds familiar. I just noticed that you just said your favorite manic statement—'Can't you just let me have some fun?' You know I want you to have fun. And you know that I want you to have a break from the depression, but you sound manic, and I have to get some help for you. Can you see that you're saying and doing all the things you do when you start to get manic? Let's take care of this now before it goes too far. I'm going to call your doctor—you told me that was okay when we discussed this before."

■ *Anxiety talking.* "I have to get out of here. I can't breathe. I feel like the walls are pressing in on me. My chest hurts! I can feel pains in my ribs! I can't breathe!"

Response. "Here, let's sit down. Breathe in as slowly as possible and then breathe out the same way. I think you're having a panic attack. You told me about these. This is a pretty crowded place and it's just too stimulating. Once your breathing is back to normal, we can leave."

Why Responding Works

When friends or family members respond to you by helping you see that bipolar disorder is talking, instead of getting into a pointless bipolar conversation, they are addressing the illness rather than what you're actually saying. If someone reacts to what you say and tells you that your life is fine when you're depressed, you can't listen. Depression won't let you listen. Responding instead of reacting gets straight to the problem and often gets through to you even when the bipolar disorder is strong. Your friends and family members need to learn to break through the language of bipolar disorder and address the real issue: that you're sick and need their help.

It's especially important that your friends and family know your leading comments and actions for mania and suicidal symptoms, as these are often the hardest issues to treat if they go too far. When your friends, family members, and health care professionals take the time to learn about this illness, they can be an invaluable tool in your healing simply because they can often see that you're sick before you can. Teach them to help you, and then promise yourself that you'll listen when they recognize the bipolar conversation and tell you that you need some help. It may be enough for your friends and family to read this chapter. They will then know what to look for. It also helps if you teach your therapist and other health care professionals this technique. One helpful exercise is to write your leading comments and actions on an index card with the solutions on the back. You can give this card to the people who help you when you're sick. This way you know that their help is coming directly from you: You wrote it when you were well for them to use when you're sick.

Paul's Story

Age 29

It took my father almost two years to learn how to talk to me when I get sick. He just couldn't separate what I said from the person I am. He always assumed that I meant everything I said. I would say, "I'm so bored with my life. I don't seem to have any direction and just wish I could know what I want to do!" He would say, "I agree. You *are* just floating through life. Why don't you get your act together and do something about your problems!" This didn't help me get better! It made me feel awful. He never really noticed that when I was stable, I never talked this way. One day I was depressed and I said, "I don't have any friends I can depend on." And he said, "I agree. I never liked your friends." He didn't pick up on the fact that I always talk this way when I'm depressed. It has nothing to do with my friends or where I am in life. I would say these things even though work was fine and I had just gone to a dinner party with all of my good friends the night before. Finally I taught him about the bipolar conversation and very, very specifically told him what I needed him to say when he hears certain leading comments and conversations. It was hard for him. He was so sure that there was something wrong with me that seeing it as an illness making me say these things seemed impossible to him. Now he knows what to look for and really helps me. When he hears me start my typical depression conversation, he says, "It sounds like you're depressed today. You always talk like this when you're depressed. What are you doing to treat the depression?" and then we talk about bipolar disorder instead of my so-called messed-up life.

■ *For Family and Friends*

You can use the following section to write your new responses to the old conversations you may have continually had with your loved one.

YOUR RESPONSES

Use the following exercise to practice what you want to say to yourself and what you want others to say to you when you're sick. After each symptom, write the language that you know will get through to you and will help you focus on treating bipolar disorder first, instead of starting a bipolar conversation.

Depression: _____

_____

_____

_____

_____

_____

Paranoia: _____

_____

_____

_____

_____

_____

Anger: _____

_____

_____

_____

_____

_____

Mania: _____

_____

_____

_____

_____

_____

_____

Anxiety: _____

_____

_____

_____

_____

_____

Learning to change your behavior surrounding what you say and do when you're in a mood swing is one of the most powerful tools you and your loved ones have to recognize, stop, and ultimately prevent the conversations that lead to anger, frustration, and broken relationships. Once you and the people around you learn to see the leading comments, the leading actions, and the resulting bipolar conversations as signs that you're getting sick, you can go into prevention mode immediately and prevent serious mood swings. It's even more effective when you can learn to recognize and do something about your own bipolar disorder leading comments and actions. You can get help much sooner than in the past. Becoming more aware of your own behavior so that you can take part in your own treatment plan takes a considerable burden off your family and friends, who will no longer have to constantly wonder what mood you're in whenever you start a conversation.

Your Toolbox

Knowledge about bipolar disorder.

A correct diagnosis.

A list of your major symptoms.

Medication knowledge.

Help with side effects.

A regular sleep schedule.

A bipolar-friendly diet.

A daily walk.

Regular and appropriate bright light exposure.

A clear picture of your work history.

A clear picture of your current financial position.

A list of your bipolar disorder triggers.

Tips to modify and stop the triggers.

The ability to recognize the bipolar conversation.

A list of leading comments and actions.

The ability to respond instead of reacting to your own bipolar disorder language.

ASKING FOR HELP

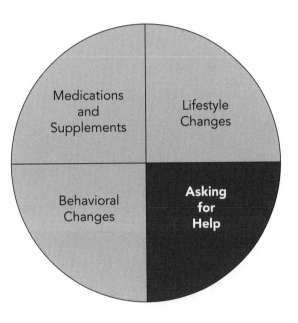

Medications and Supplements

Lifestyle Changes

Behavioral Changes

Asking for Help

CHAPTER 6

CHOOSING A SUPPORTIVE HEALTH CARE TEAM

The final and very important step in your 4-Step Plan is finding the right people to help you instead of just taking what you are given once you are diagnosed with bipolar disorder. If you spend more time selecting fruit at a grocery store than choosing a supportive health care provider, you are not alone. Many people are so used to insurance companies and hospitals making their choices for them, they forget that ultimately they are the ones who decide the quality of the health care they receive. You *do* have the power to choose the health care team you feel will fit your needs. You have the ability to educate yourself on what works for you and then go out and find the people to help you create and maintain stability.

As you know, because bipolar disorder is such a highly complex illness, the most effective way to treat it successfully is to approach it from many different angles. One of the best ways to do this is to create a supportive health care team that fits your various needs.

■ *For Family and Friends*

You may be the one who helps your loved one pick a health care team. Depending on how ill a person is—especially someone recently out of the hospital—family members are often the only people to advocate for appropriate health care. It helps if you take the ideas in this chapter into account so that your loved one is satisfied with the health care team when he or she is again well enough to take charge of treatment.

Why You Need a Supportive Health Care Team

Bipolar disorder needs to be managed daily. When you have the help of a team who's on your side, your chances for stability are greatly enhanced. It's estimated that 15 to 20 percent of people with *untreated* mood disorders will commit suicide, but that number is significantly smaller among those who are treated for bipolar disorder with a comprehensive plan.[1] A supportive health care team is one of the main resources people with bipolar disorder need for this comprehensive plan.

When you were first diagnosed with bipolar disorder and realized that your illness requires lifetime management, there's a good chance you were stunned. If you're like most people, you were sent home with a bag of pills and an appointment sometime in the future. You were then left alone to process the information. You may have felt scared, intimidated, or confused by your appointment. After you got home, you probably thought of all the questions you wished you had asked.

Or maybe you were given the diagnosis after a traumatic hospital stay. It can be hard to think of how you will possibly manage bipolar disorder effectively when you're experiencing so many emotions. Yet even in your most desperate times, help is available. This chapter will teach you to take charge and choose a team to help you manage this illness so that you can find stability and get back to your life. The goal is to help you get clear on exactly what you want from your health care team and to then give you the tools you need to search for, interview, and ultimately choose that team.

■ *For Family and Friends*

When your loved one is first diagnosed with bipolar disorder, it helps if you have a list of questions ready for his or her health care professionals. You can ask, "What role will I have to play in helping my loved one find stability? What are my rights as a family member or friend?" Write down what you want to say and ask before you see a health care professional.

WHY YOU NEED A HEALTH CARE *TEAM*

Many people with bipolar disorder feel overwhelmed and inadvertently ruin their relationships by needing too much from too few people. They often have one doctor whom they see maybe once a month, and then depend on friends and family for the rest of the considerable support they need. Have you ever felt that your needs regarding this illness are just too big for the people in your life to handle? Then you're not alone. When you create a team of people to help you find and maintain stability, you can spread your needs among many people so that you can maintain and nurture all your relationships successfully, with minimum stress.

The Many Faces of Your Health Care Team

A medications doctor is of course an essential part of any health care team, but if you want to manage this illness successfully, you'll need a lot more support than someone you see, at most, once a week. There are many people you can look to for help in managing bipolar disorder, from a close friend or trusted colleague to a therapist or naturopath. The first step of the process is deciding on the qualities you want the people on your team to possess. When you're clear on what you want, it becomes easier for you to attract people to your team. Look over the following list and check the qualities you feel are important for the people on your health care team.

Qualities You Are Looking For in a Health Care Provider

- ☐ Someone who listens.
- ☐ A physical health expert.
- ☐ Help with medication management.
- ☐ Someone who truly understands bipolar disorder.
- ☐ Someone who understands my own symptoms.
- ☐ Nonjudgmental care.
- ☐ Tolerance.
- ☐ Someone who keeps a cool head in an emergency.
- ☐ Someone who offers specific tips I can use to stay stable.

- ☐ Tough love.
- ☐ Someone who tells it like it is.
- ☐ A friend.
- ☐ A mentor.
- ☐ Someone fun.
- ☐ A teacher.
- ☐ Someone who will not lie to me even when it hurts.
- ☐ Someone to ease me into change.
- ☐ Male.
- ☐ Female.
- ☐ Someone with the time to help comprehensively.
- ☐ A provider covered by insurance.
- ☐ Someone free to spend time with me.
- ☐ A compassionate person.
- ☐ A harsh taskmaster.
- ☐ Someone who offers concrete suggestions.
- ☐ Someone who can provide the safety needed to talk about scary things.
- ☐ Someone I can cry with.
- ☐ Someone willing to try new treatments.

It's important that you're clear on the qualities that work for you. Do you want your team members to be gentle friends or people who can be aggressive and forceful in your health care? Do you want someone who is compassionate and loving or do you prefer someone who is more into constructive criticism and tells it like it is? Maybe you need a little of both. It's essential that you make these decisions for yourself when you're relatively stable, because these are the people who will help you when you're ill. Remember, if you don't make these decisions for yourself, someone else will be forced to make them for you.

Once you've decided on the qualities you want in the people on your team, you can get specific and choose people who meet your needs. The following table takes the qualities listed above and matches them to the health care professionals, friends, and family members you may want on your team.

CREATING YOUR HEALTH CARE TEAM

Quality	Role/Title of Person
Someone to listen to me	Therapist, naturopath, friend, family member, doctor, psychiatrist, support group, Web forum.
Physical health	Primary care physician, naturopath, dentist, chiropractor, acupuncturist, nurse practitioner, massage therapist, yoga teacher, meditation teacher, personal trainer, martial arts teacher, anyone else who works on the body.
Help with medication management	Psychiatrist, nurse practitioner, primary care physician.
Compassion/understanding	Therapist, naturopath, support group, nurse practitioner, friend, family member, psychiatrist, primary care physician.
Someone who understands bipolar disorder	Support group, specialized health care practitioner, Web forum, friend with bipolar disorder.
Nonjudgmental care	Naturopath, therapist, compassionate health care professional, carefully chosen friends, family members, co-workers.
Practical advice	Psychiatrist, therapist, pragmatic health care professional, someone who manages the illness successfully, mentor, others who have experienced serious illness.
Tolerance	Choose people who naturally have this quality.
Time	Naturopath, therapist, support group, psychiatrist or general doctor in private practice, Web forum.
Specific tips I can use to stay stable	Therapist trained in bipolar disorder treatment, monitored support group, Web pages, this book, national and local mental health organizations.

As you can see, you have many options regarding the people you choose. The point of this exercise is for you to broaden your expectations so that you can include more people on your health care team instead of relying on one doctor and your friends and family exclusively. When you actively participate in choosing your team, you take charge of bipolar disorder and learn to manage the illness on *your* terms. This is a powerful way to create stability in your life and work toward preventing mood swings.

The following section will help you create your personal health care team. Look over the list of health care professionals below and put a check next to the ones you would like on your team. You can then decide how to find these professionals if you do not already see them regularly. The point is that you are far more in control of who you see and the type of care you receive from health care professionals than you may realize. You have more options than just seeing someone to check your medications.

Your Health Care Team

☐ Psychiatrist
☐ General practitioner
☐ Chiropractor
☐ Dentist
☐ Compassionate friends
☐ Co-workers I can trust
☐ Web forum

☐ Naturopath
☐ Therapist
☐ Massage therapist
☐ Personal trainer
☐ Family members who want to help
☐ Monitored support group

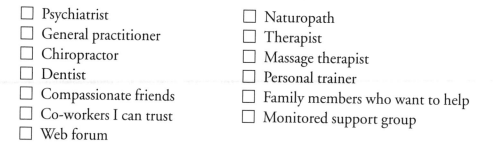

Include a Dentist on Your Team

Many people with bipolar disorder have trouble with their teeth due to medication side effects (one theory is that the dry mouth caused by many medications causes teeth to become brittle), grinding teeth at night, clenching and cracking teeth, and the overall stress of going through mood swings. Try to visit your dentist regularly and prevent these expensive and painful problems.

Asking for a Referral

Now that you have a better idea of the people you want on your side, you're ready to get started on your quest for the team that will help you find and maintain stability. One of the best ways to do this is to ask friends, family members, and your current health care team members for referrals. Ask them about the quality of the care they receive, then use their information to help you make informed decisions.

As with all decisions, there are some logistical questions you need to ask about your health care professionals as well:

- Is the care cost-effective?
- Is the person accepted by my insurance?
- How long does it take to get an appointment?
- What if I have an emergency?
- What if I need to go to the hospital?
- Do I need a referral?
- Is seeing this person financially feasible—not just now but in the future as well?
- What are my options if I have no money or insurance?

Choosing Your Psychiatric Medications Doctor

One of the most important members of your health care team is the person who will pre-scribe and monitor your medications. You have a few options when you choose this per-son. Traditionally, the work was done by a psychiatrist, but times have changed, and many people are now seen and monitored by their general practitioner. Although the National Institute of Mental Health says, "While primary-care physicians who do not specialize in psychiatry also may prescribe these medications, it's recommended that people with bipolar disorder see a psychiatrist for treatment,"[2] there is a good chance you will have to use a general doctor for your medication monitoring. The best choice is a psy-chiatrist, especially when you are first diagnosed, but rest assured that other health care professionals, if carefully chosen, can provide excellent medication care as well. Here are some ideas on the qualities to look for in your medications doctor:

- Understands the illness.
- Has time for me, listens to me.
- Keeps up to date on the latest medications.

- Is willing to work to find the right combination of medications.
- Understands the impact that side effects have on my life.
- Is clearly committed to doing what it takes to help me find stability.
- Has ideas on resources that would give me additional help.
- Is open to comprehensive treatment and offers ideas on how I can manage the illness at home.

The point of this section is to get you to think of your health care team in a professional way. You're the employer. You're the one with the choices. Think of yourself as a manager hiring a staff. You are the person paying for this service. The more aware you become of what you want and need, the better your chance of finding stability.

The following questions can help you get clear on what you want from your medications doctor. If you already have a doctor, you can use these questions to learn more about his or her background and treatment philosophy.

- Does the person take time to talk with patients? Does he or she explain what is involved in the diagnosis and treatment of bipolar disorder?
- Does the person understand the physical issues you may have due to mood swings and medications?
- Does the person talk in a language you understand? Do you feel you are working together as a team? Do you feel listened to, understood, and respected?
- Does the person understand that bipolar disorder affects your personal life as well, and that you need help in that area?
- Does the person emphasize wellness and self-care by encouraging you to take charge of your own healing process so that you can find physical health and mental stability?
- Is the person open to your supplementing more traditional treatments with complementary treatments?
- Can you reach the person at night or on weekends in case of an emergency?

Asking these questions and carefully considering the answers you receive can help you decide on a medications doctor who meets your specific needs. In fact, you can and should use these questions for every health care professional on your team. What matters is that you're now thinking ahead and becoming an active participant in your health care instead of just taking on someone at random. You're becoming a manager.

Once you find a person you would like to work with, you can be ready with some interview questions that will give you insight into his or her philosophy and help you get a feel for him or her as a person. Here are some suggestions:

- How much experience do you have with bipolar disorder?
- Are you familiar with the latest medications?
- What are your ideas on treating this illness successfully?
- Can you tell me a little bit about yourself, where you went to school, and what your treatment philosophy is?
- What is your philosophy on complementary treatments?

If your prospective or current doctor gets defensive about these questions or brushes them away as unimportant, this is a sign you can't ignore. There can be many reasons for defensiveness. Your doctor may be burned out by the system, or it may be a personality issue. A poor response to your questions may be a sign that your future together may have some problems. If you have the option of another doctor, you may want to make a change. You have a right and an obligation to ask these questions and to be taken seriously. The good news is that most doctors will willingly answer your questions, and you can create a better relationship by knowing a bit more about them.

Your medications doctor needs to be someone you can talk with easily. Considering that bipolar disorder is an illness that requires daily medical treatment and monitoring, it's very important that you have a medications doctor you like and respect—someone compassionate and understanding. If you're scared or intimidated by this person, it can affect the outcome of your treatment.

When You Want to Change Doctors

Maybe after going through the exercises in this chapter, you feel it's time to change your current doctor to someone who better meets your needs. You may need more quality time or compassion, or maybe there is simply a personality clash. This is normal and nothing to be ashamed of. It doesn't mean your doctor isn't a good doctor, but simply that he or she is not the best doctor for you. It can be intimidating to see someone you don't connect with, and it certainly doesn't help you find stability. It may be that you can simply call your doctor's office and ask to see someone new. Your insurance company can help you with this as well. Also, there is always the reality that your medications doctor has *very* limited time to see you. This means you will have to get your needs met from other health care professionals.

What to Do if You Can't Change Doctors

If you're unhappy with your health care but can't change the people you see for financial or insurance reasons, then it's time for you to try to change the way your doctor interacts with you. Be honest and tell him or her in realistic and reasonable terms what you need. Be calm and professional and tell the doctor you believe he or she can provide better health care. It may be that the doctor is just simply tired and has forgotten how important a personal touch is. You can be the one to remind your doctor that you need compassion.

Adam's Story

Age 20

When I was diagnosed, I knew nothing. I assumed that the doctors knew exactly what they were doing and that all would be just fine! My first state-supplied doctor was too busy to help and too old to care. I know that's harsh. But I was sick and neither the doctor nor social worker had time for me. Then something happened. I got a doctor who somehow managed to look at me and say, "How are you?" and really mean it. I'm not sure if a doctor had really looked at me until then. I said, "I'm not doing very well," and started to cry. He gave me some tissues, opened my file, and said, "Let's see what we can do about that." He doesn't have a lot of time, either, but the time we have together means something. We get things done. All because he learned how to keep his empathy while still being busy. I am sure he got frustrated with me or scared when I was so suicidal or when I once called him in a manic episode and told him I was cured, but he never showed it. He is the reason I kept trying new medications and started to change my lifestyle. He gave me books to read and encouraged me to challenge my own bipolar thoughts. I am as stable as I can be right now because he believed in me.

You can be honest and tell him or her that you feel rushed and worried after an appointment, and then ask for your doctor's ideas on how you can both improve the situation. This will at least start a discussion between you. The following suggestions can help you talk with your doctor if you're not pleased with your health care:

- I often feel stressed because we have so little time to talk about my treatment. Do you have any suggestions on how to improve this?
- I need more help with this illness. Do you have any suggestions?
- I know that you're very busy, but I need to know the ideas you have on how I can treat this illness more effectively.

You always have the option of telling your health care professional what you're really thinking. This is much better than going home stressed and worried about your treatment future. Doctors are invaluable members of your health care team. The better you interact, the better chance you have to remain stable.

Reminding Yourself to Be Reasonable

It can be difficult to step outside yourself, especially when you're frustrated at the quality of care you're receiving. But it's important to consider that your doctor is a human being just like you, with the stresses and problems of anyone trying to help many people with serious illnesses in a very short amount of time. Practicing this kind of tolerance can take all your energy, which is why it's essential that you make your health care decisions when you're relatively stable. If you react and fire your doctor because of a bipolar disorder mood swing, you will regret it later. The first step is to try to work things out with the doctor you currently have. It's always a challenge to be open and ready to accept the care your team member has to offer you, while also being ready to stick up for what you need. This may take practice, but you can learn to do it.

CHOOSING A THERAPIST

Now that you're thinking about the type of medications doctor you want on your team, you can use the same process to find a therapist. A therapist who understands or who *is willing to learn about bipolar disorder* can be invaluable. Because bipolar disorder has symptoms that seem very psychological and emotional, it's essential that you educate the therapist you choose on what it's like to have mood swings. Your therapist can learn when to talk about problems that are real and when to talk about treating bipolar disorder specifically. It helps if you can tell your therapist what to look for when you're sick. The following script will give you an idea of how to educate your therapist about bipolar disorder and how it affects your view on life:

> I cry a lot when I'm in a downswing. It doesn't mean my life is terrible; it just means I'm sick and need to focus on taking care of the depression. When I'm slightly manic, I talk really fast and seem very excited. I jump into new situations without thinking, and rarely think things through to the end result. This doesn't mean that we need to address my desire to do too much. Instead, we need to address the mania. I need suggestions on how to prevent the mania instead of a discussion on what I'm doing wrong in my life because of the mania.
>
> You may notice that there are some days when I'm unnaturally upset about my life even though I was just fine the week before. This probably makes you think that I'm really unhappy about something and that we have to dig deep to find the causes of my unhappiness. The truth is that bipolar disorder often makes me upset about my life. It tells me that my life is pointless and worthless. This is part of the illness. It's very important that you ask me if I'm in a mood swing when we meet, especially if you notice that I'm different from the last time we

A Note on Money

Money will always play a role in your health care decisions, but don't let it make those decisions for you. Be firm in your needs and ask for what you want. If you can't pay, ask if there are other options available. Look into bartering, discounts, and scholarships. You can always ask a health care professional about your options. You can also join a Web forum, read books, and visit self-help groups that offer concrete suggestions on getting better. The point is, do everything you can to find the help you need when money is an issue. As you use the tips in this book and become more stable, there's a good chance that you can improve your financial situation.

met. We can then talk about managing this illness instead of dwelling on what bipolar disorder is telling me is wrong with my life. I'm working hard on learning to manage my mood swings and I need your help with this.

In the space provided below, write what you would like to tell your therapist about bipolar disorder and how it affects your behavior when you're in a session.

_____

_____

_____

_____

_____

Talking together about bipolar disorder can lessen your therapist's confusion over your behavior and will educate him or her on the role that bipolar disorder plays in your life. Therapy can be a very important part of your healing process, but if it addresses the issues and behaviors caused by bipolar disorder as something psychological instead of physical symptoms of an illness, progress can be slow. Once you teach your therapist what is real and what is the illness, you can truly make some amazing progress.

The following section explores some of your options regarding the psychotherapy used to treat bipolar disorder.

DOES PSYCHOTHERAPY WORK?

Several types of psychotherapy have documented success in treating bipolar disorder—always in combination with medication treatment. Not all forms of psychotherapy are effective for bipolar disorder, so it's important that you inquire about specific expertise a therapist has with any of the following treatment approaches:

- *Individual or family psychoeducational therapy.* Here the focus is largely educational, helping the patient and his or her family members understand the illness, medications, side effects, illness management, and relapse prevention. What is especially helpful is working with family members to help them notice what may be the early

Sarah's Story (Psychotherapist)

Age 60

When I started working with people who had bipolar disorder, I have to admit I had my own ideas on what was wrong with them. Yes, *wrong*. I really believed that bipolar came from some kind of unresolved childhood trauma. This was years ago. Many therapists believed this. The parents must have done something. Then as I watched my clients struggle with the same issues I really realized that my methods weren't working. Having someone talk about their so-called problems simply doesn't work if the problems stem from an illness. One of my clients is literally a different person each time she comes in the office. I would wonder, *Who will I see today? The confident person who has no worries? The anxious person that rocks a bit as she talks and keeps rubbing her hands and eyes? Or the one who cries through the whole session?* The more I thought about it, the easier it was to see that *she* was not changing from session to session. Her outward mood and behaviors were changing. If we talked about the bipolar and not what the bipolar was saying, we actually got somewhere. She could say, "I know this is not the real me talking. The real me feels this . . . the bipolar me says this." It was a breakthrough for me, as I now understand what she really needs and not what it seems like she needs.

signs of a newly emerging mood swing. It is always critical to notice such early signs, and often loved ones notice these before they are recognized by the individual with bipolar disorder. Typically, this type of therapy averages seven sessions, and has been shown in research to significantly reduce the frequency of relapses and to improve quality of life.[3]

- *Family therapy.* In addition to psychoeducation regarding illness, this form of intervention also coaches the patient and family members in improving communication conflict-resolution, and problem-solving skills. This form of treatment is also well supported by research.[4]
- *Cognitive therapy.* This approach teaches effective coping skills, and it, too, has a track record of effectiveness.[5] The main thrust of cognitive therapy is to teach skills

in clear thinking and problem solving—specifically, dealing with unreasonable and often very painful thoughts by examining them for veracity and then replacing them with more realistic and reasonable thoughts.

■ *Listening/talk therapy* can be invaluable for treating bipolar disorder if done by someone who truly understands your needs and the symptoms of bipolar disorder.

You now have some ideas on how to choose the medications doctor and the therapist you want on your team. You can use the previous examples to make careful decisions regarding all the people you see.

EDUCATING YOUR TEAM ON WHAT YOU NEED

Once you have decided on a health care team, the next step is to teach yourself how to tell them what you need. Many people with bipolar disorder simply assume that the people whom they depend on for help will know what they need. Not so: All members of your health care team, even those trained to work with patients, need specific guidance. The illness can appear very random and chaotic to people on the outside (even for those who work with bipolar disorder), and knowing what to do may feel impossible for some of the health care professionals you see. *You* may understand the difference between anxiety, depression, irritation, and mania, for example, but the people in your life and especially those on your health care team need to know exactly what you're experiencing so that you can get the help you need.

One way to do this is to simply tell people what's going on. When you see your doctor, you can say, "I'm depressed today and I'm working on it. I'm sure I'll talk like a depressed person." When you're slightly manic and have to see your therapist, you can say, "I'm probably going to talk way too fast today. Can you help me with this?" It helps if you stay focused on the practical. Try to be clear on what helps and what doesn't help, and let people know exactly what you need during the appointment.

Communicating with Your Team

Once you choose a medications doctor and your other health care professionals, you may still have quite a few communication problems. Appointments can feel very rushed. You may forget what you want to ask and, as almost always happens with medical doctors, you may feel pressured to say everything you need to say in a short period of time. One way to get around this is to think carefully about your appointment before you get there. You can write down the questions you want to ask and get clear on the exact help you need before you get to the office. In other words, you can do the homework needed so that your appointments can be successful. The following section of this chapter is designed to help you make all of your appointments more effective.

Once you have chosen a health care professional, you can focus on your next appointment. Use the following checklist to get ready:

- [ ] Take this book with you to all appointments.
- [ ] Take a calendar to all appointments.
- [ ] Think of the questions you want to ask and write them down.
- [ ] Write down all of the topics you want to cover.
- [ ] Make a list of what you need to take with you, including any needed paperwork.
- [ ] Write down any medication needs or questions you have.
- [ ] Make sure you're clear on the length of the appointment and that you use your time wisely.
- [ ] If the appointment is in a new location, check on parking and driving directions, and plan accordingly in order to reduce your stress.
- [ ] Create a file that includes all of this information. You can carry it with you to the appointment and then add any new paperwork you receive. (See chapter 9.)

Careful preparation is essential if you want to maximize the help you receive in your appointments.

MANAGING BIPOLAR DISORDER BETWEEN APPOINTMENTS

When your next doctor's appointment seems too far away, you can become overly stressed and worried about your health. This is when you have to take charge of your own health care and use the other people on your team to help you stay well. Who else on your team can you ask for help when you can't see your doctor? How can you take steps to take care of yourself between health care visits?

Effective Communication During Appointments

- Know what you want to say before you get to your appointment.
- Remember that your health care provider is human.
- Be honest about your feelings, but make sure that you're not letting the bipolar disorder talk for you.
- Make the best use of your time.
- Let the person you're seeing know if you're in a mood swing. It's okay if you cry, but the more stable you can be, the better.

Remember, bipolar disorder is an illness, it's not the real you. You have to separate yourself from the symptoms when you have a long time to wait between doctor's visits. You have to work on yourself and do what you can to help yourself find stability. If you agree that managing this illness is not only about medications, then it makes sense that there are many things you can do between doctor's visits to stay well. If there's an emergency, then get more immediate help, but if not, you will have to learn to break your dependence on your doctor. Your doctor is an important tool in your management, but you're actually the biggest part of your team.

This book offers many ideas on what to do between doctor's visits. Once you practice these management skills, the time between appointments can feel less stressful. One way to do this is to create a list of what you can do to take care of yourself between visits.

When you're feeling sick and can't see your medications doctor, what steps can you take to find help? List your options here. Some examples have been added.

Think of what I can do for myself first.
Talk with a trusted friend.
Call my therapist.
Read this book.
See a naturopath.
Go to a support group.

_____

_____

_____

_____

_____

BEING CAREFUL NOT TO EXPECT TOO MUCH FROM OTHERS

By now you have assembled or are working on assembling a strong support system of health care professionals. However, never forget your own central role in managing this illness. Ultimately, it's up to you. If you always look to yourself first and do what you can to manage the bipolar disorder comprehensively by using the tips from your health care team and those covered in this book, then you will be able to ask for help when you really need it instead of overwhelming the people in your life with excessive neediness. You really are your best advocate and are definitely the most important part of your health care team. Don't forget yourself and the important role you play in your own health care.

CREATING A BRIGHTER FUTURE

You won't regret taking the time to choose your health care team carefully. Always remember that when you need to ask for help, you do have the right and the skills to find the team that will work best for you. This is your life. Choose the health care team you feel will work the best for you. Remember that these people may be in your life for years. They will be there when you're manic, depressed, psychotic, anxious, obsessive, suicidal,

■ *For Family and Friends*

What role can you play on your loved one's health care team? It may be you don't want to play the caretaker role, or maybe that is your natural personality. Tell the person what you want to and can do. Be honest. If you are a friend, the friendship will suffer if you aren't honest. If someone is overwhelming you, tell him or her in a kind way and suggest what you need. It's better than losing your relationship.

or physically sick. It's a good idea to take time and put a lot of thought into who you want on your team. Chapter 7 will help you apply these ideas to the friends and family members you want to ask for help and support. Always choose the people on your team carefully. You are worth it.

Your Toolbox

Knowledge about bipolar disorder.

A correct diagnosis.

A list of your major symptoms.

Medication knowledge.

Help with side effects.

A regular sleep schedule.

A bipolar-friendly diet.

A daily walk.

Regular and appropriate bright light exposure.

A clear picture of your work history.

A clear picture of your current financial position.

A list of your bipolar disorder triggers.

Tips to modify and stop the triggers.

The ability to recognize the bipolar conversation.

A list of leading comments and actions.

The ability to respond instead of reacting to your own bipolar disorder language.

A supportive health care team.

Well-planned appointments.

CHAPTER 7

TEACHING FAMILY AND FRIENDS HOW TO HELP YOU STAY STABLE

Have you noticed that asking for help from family members and friends can strain your relationships—especially if you are really sick and needy? This is common because bipolar disorder, and especially untreated bipolar disorder, is an illness that burdens and often ruins relationships. It's normal if you feel confused, scared, and hopeless when it comes to treating this illness. Sometimes the amount of help you need can feel overwhelming. One way you may deal with these feelings is to blindly ask the people in your life for help, but problems can arise if you ask the wrong people or overwhelm a few people with your needs.

This chapter will help you get clear on what information your friends and family members need and want to know about bipolar disorder. It will teach you how to choose the right friends and family to join your health care team, and will then show you how to teach these people what works and what doesn't work to help you stay stable. In reality, most people have no idea how to help someone with bipolar disorder, and you can become frustrated and saddened by what seems like a lack of caring. The goal of this chapter is to help you organize

> ■ *For Family and Friends*
>
> You often play a far more significant role in your loved one's life than his or her health care professionals. This can be quite a burden—but it can also be a positive if you and your loved one can review this chapter together and learn new ways of working with each other to manage the illness.

what you can do to involve your friends and family in your bipolar disorder treatment plan so that you get the help you need without overwhelming or scaring the people you love.

UNDERSTANDING WHY THIS ILLNESS IS SO HARD ON RELATIONSHIPS

It's natural that when you feel sick, you want to turn to your friends and family for help. The problem is that just because people are friends or relatives, it doesn't mean they're necessarily the right people to turn to when you're ill. When you ask for help from people who are either not capable or not willing to do what you ask, it can lead to anger, frustration, and relationship problems all around. The solution is learning to help yourself more effectively first and then turning to friends and family members with specific requests that take into account their ability and desire to help you. You really can learn to ask for help from the right people, spread that request for help among many people, and keep your relationships strong and intact.

Taking charge of bipolar disorder takes a lot of work. You often need so much help that it may seem impossible to get what you need from your doctor and other health care professionals. As you read in chapter 6, the team approach works well because this illness is so complex and often overwhelming. One way to smooth your treatment path is to make sure the people around you are very clear about what this illness means and how it affects your life. Their reaction to this information will help you choose those you want on your health care team and educate them about the reality of bipolar disorder.

HOW TO TALK TO YOUR FRIENDS AND FAMILY ABOUT BIPOLAR DISORDER

What do you think your friends and family members need to know about bipolar disorder? Maybe they're confused and have no idea what you're going through. Maybe they think you just have "problems" that you can't or won't control. One way to deal with this issue is to ask them to read this book and come to you with any questions they have about the illness. It's also a good idea to create a set explanation for the illness that is easy to understand and that can be used in any situation. You can then sit down with friends and family, clearly explain the illness, and tell them what you need. The next step is to ask if they have any questions about what you just explained.

Questions from Friends and Family Members

What are some of the questions your friends and family members have about bipolar disorder? Have you asked them what they want to know? This is a good time to sit down with them and say, "It must be scary for you to know that I have this illness. What questions do you have about the diagnosis and my behavior?" You may be surprised at the questions they ask. You can then talk together about their fears and worries, and get bipolar disorder out in the open as an illness instead of something you do wrong.

Here are some tips for talking with friends and family about bipolar disorder:

- Define bipolar disorder clearly.
- Explain how it affects your life.
- Tell them how you feel about having the illness.
- Explain that your behaviors are sometimes controlled by bipolar disorder and are not done on purpose.
- Ask them to read this book.
- Ask for their questions, write them down, and answer them as best you can.

Write the questions from your friends and family here:

_____

_____

_____

_____

_____

_____

_____

_____

_____

_____

The Difficult Questions and Comments

How many times have you heard people say, "Why can't you just get it together and live like a normal person?" How often do people tell you to just snap out of it and not be so emotional? These are typical reactions from people who don't understand the illness. Now that you have more background on why you act the way you do, you can start to teach the people in your life about bipolar disorder and why it affects your emotions and behaviors

---

Tawnya's Story

Age 25

I heard some really rotten stuff when I was first diagnosed. It was as though some people thought I had leprosy. Did people think they were going to catch something from me? Some of my friends never came back. It was the ones I used to party with. I couldn't have kept up with them anymore anyway. The friends that did stay were a bit clueless. They would ask me if I was okay or if I needed anything. They knew I was very embarrassed about what I did when I was so depressed. A few saw me in restraints because the doctors thought I would hurt myself. It's like someone seeing you drunk and throwing up. I'm not sure it's an image they will ever forget. I decided to be honest about it all. I had been hiding things for so long, I couldn't hide the bipolar stuff anymore. I was always a really independent friend. I never stayed in one place for long and I was not too dependable. When I got out the hospital, I needed a lot more from people. It's as though the meds gave me the ability to say, "I need help or I won't make it." My family is not really around much, so my friends are the ones who help me. I was on disability for a while, so they bought dinners and stuff. When they see me down they say, "Are you sick today?" instead of the normal, "What's wrong?" The answer to that question is always, "Bipolar is what's wrong! I hate it!" I now work at a coffee shop. Not exactly the high life I used to live before. I think that trying to kill myself ended my old life. I'm glad I have friends. I must have done something right before because so many of them stuck around. I am quite happy now. I don't think about death all the time anymore.

so strongly. It helps if you have set answers ready for the tough questions. Remember, the people who ask these questions are not necessarily trying to hurt you. They simply don't understand the illness, and it's up to you to educate them so that they can help you instead of upsetting you.

Here are some of the tough questions and comments you may have to deal with. Put a check next to each question or comment you've heard. Add your own experiences to the end of the list.

- What's wrong with you?
- Why are you sick all the time?
- When are you going to get better?
- Why do you spend so much money when you're sick?
- What did you do to catch this illness?
- Why are you so emotional?
- I bet you could deal with this if you just tried harder.
- Everyone else can work; why can't you?
- Why are you so weird?
- You could do so much if you would just settle down.
- I don't understand you at all.
- Do you want to ruin your life?

Write some of the difficult questions and comments you have heard here:

_____

_____

_____

_____

_____

How to Respond to the Tough Questions and Comments

The more you can learn to respond to what people say instead of reacting to how the questions and comments make you feel, the more effectively you can explain this illness to your friends and family members. Even though you may be hurt and angry by the in-

■ *For Family and Friends*

There is no need to feel guilty if you have asked any of the questions listed here. Most family members and friends are frustrated by bipolar disorder behavior that just makes no sense. If your loved one was diagnosed later in life, you may have been asking these questions for years. That is okay. It happens. You now know that the questions and comments are pointless. You can learn new and more helpful responses to your loved one's behavior.

sensitivity of others, it always helps if you acknowledge their questions and comments and then give your responses calmly and clearly.

Read over the following examples of how you can respond to some of the difficult questions and comments you may hear. After the examples, there is space for you to write your own replies:

- ■ I know you think I can't control myself sometimes. I understand that's how I appear to you. If I had leukemia or diabetes, would you ask me why I can't control my white blood cells or my insulin? Bipolar disorder is a physical illness that affects my brain chemistry—this then affects my emotions. If you can accept that, you can understand why I have trouble. I know my behavior is often weird. I'm working on it. This behavior is a symptom for most people with bipolar disorder. If you can help me get more stable, the weird behavior will get better as well.
- ■ Many people with bipolar disorder have trouble with work. Work's a very stimulating place and, as you know, I have trouble when I get overstimulated. My brain responds differently than other brains. I need your help in figuring out what I can do to support myself so that I can be more productive.
- ■ I'm not like most other people, because I have an illness. But I am like the other people with bipolar disorder. I'm just not like you because you don't have bipolar disorder. Can you accept me for how I am and read this book with me so that we can manage the illness together?
- ■ One of the symptoms of mania, as strange as it seems, is spending money. It's a well-documented symptom. When I get manic, I spend without thinking. I really need your help to monitor my spending so that mania doesn't wreck my finances.

■ Bipolar disorder is an illness that makes me respond to outside events with way over-the-top reactions. You may go through the same event and have a normal reaction because your brain is normal. My brain can't do this as well as yours can. My brain creates false emotions that are often very confusing and upsetting. It's not something I do on purpose. I'm not weak and I don't have personality problems. I have an illness that makes it look like I have emotional issues—but I don't. I just have a brain that doesn't react to things correctly. I'm working to fix this by taking medications and starting the ideas in this book. Would you like to help me with this?

What would you like to say to the people who ask the difficult questions and make judgmental comments?

_____

_____

_____

_____

_____

_____

_____

■ *For Family and Friends*

Fill out the preceding section with what you want to say to people on the outside who have judged your loved one. Were you blamed for his or her behavior? Did anyone say you just needed more control over your loved one? Have you ever been too embarrassed to explain bipolar disorder to people who don't understand what your loved one is going through? This is your chance to plan what you will say the next time someone says something ignorant or unkind to you.

Michael's Story

Age 40

I can tell you that watching your child suffer from bipolar illness is one of the worst things you'll ever go through. But I can also admit that it's not as bad as I thought it was going to be when there is a realistic treatment system in place. Once the family learned more about the illness, we were not so hard on her. I remember when my sister heard about the bipolar disorder and said to my daughter, "I'm glad you're finally going to do something about your problems and do something with your life." I just wanted to go after her and choke her. I'm not kidding! This is my sister! She said this to the niece she loved and yet she had no understanding of what she was really going through. I'm not sure she even read a book or asked questions about what bipolar is. She just said what she was thinking. This has been an education process for all of us. My daughter is good at telling people how to help her, but when she gets depressed (and she is depressed *so* much less now) I do find that I have to be the one to say, "This is an illness. She is not doing anything wrong. She's not lazy. Here is what she needs." And then I teach them what my daughter has told me works when she's sick. I'm so proud of my daughter. She's not a failure because she was sick for so many years. She's a true success story in my eyes.

As you can see, there are many ways to deflate and deflect the unthinking and often judgmental questions and comments you get from the people in your life. Remind yourself that they often ask these questions out of ignorance, and may not ever understand what you go through, but at least you now know how to talk to them. Try to step outside yourself and look at your behavior from their point of view. Most people outside bipolar disorder just want to know what it means when you're sick. What does it feel like? What do you go through? And many want to know what they can do to help. Educate your friends and family members, but remember that there's no way they can understand this complex and very confusing illness unless you teach them what they need to know about their behavior toward you. One way to do this is to create a list of what you want and need to give them. It can be hard to talk about these things, but writing and reading them can make things easier.

What you want to tell your friends and family:

- Understand that I'm really trying to control the bipolar disorder, but sometimes it wins and I really can't help my behavior when I have a serious mood swing. The solution is for me to prevent the mood swings. I could use your help with this.
- Please, please remain objective and don't judge me by what I do when I'm ill. Help me to learn ways not to do the behaviors, but don't get caught up in them. Please don't punish me for being sick!
- Try not to get caught up in my mood swings and take the things I say so personally. Learn to recognize them and then use the techniques in this book to help me get well.
- Ask me what I'm going through. Don't simply ask me how I am. I'll probably lie to you. I can't be honest when I'm ill. Ask me specific questions such as "Are you psychotic now?" Or "Are you thinking of killing yourself?" Or "It seems like you're depressed; I'm going to_____. Will this help?" When I'm sick, it's hard to make healthy decisions. I really need your help when I'm sick.

Add your ideas here on what you want to tell your friends and family members when you're sick and need help:

_____

_____

_____

_____

_____

_____

_____

_____

_____

_____

■ *For Family and Friends*

What do you need to hear from your loved one? What would help your pain and worry? What explanations do you need? You can use the following section to write your hopes of what you want your loved one to say to you regarding his or her behavior during episodes of the illness. As a friend, what do you need to know and what do you need to hear? If your loved one is stable, it is completely appropriate for you to discuss what *you* need and how you can better work together to manage the illness.

DECIDING WHO CAN HELP

Getting the illness out in the open and talking with your friends and family members is a good first step to opening up communication about bipolar disorder. This will give you an idea which people are willing to at least try to understand the illness. You can then decide which people in your life can take the next step and actually help you to manage the symptoms. Friends and family members can be an essential part of your health care team, but it's very important that you choose them as carefully as you choose your health care professionals. Just because someone loves you it doesn't mean that he or she is willing or emotionally equipped to help you stay stable. If you can accept this from the beginning of your diagnosis, it will save you a lot of trouble in the future. Your relatives and closest friends all have their own lives with their own issues, and it's often too much for them to take on your illness as well. As you become clearer on what you need, and start to create a health care team, you may find that some unexpected people in your life are willing to take on the roles you were hoping certain close friends and family members would play. Your goal is to find the people who want to help, ask them what they're willing to do, and then teach them how to help you.

The following exercise will help you to decide which friends and family members you want to turn to for help as you create your health care team. As you complete this exercise, think of the people who have actually asked you how you are and meant it. Who has asked what they can do? Who calls or writes and asks how you are? Who learns about the illness and wants to know more so that they can help you? Is there an unexpected person at work who has shown an interest in what you're going through? Is there someone you hardly know who has experience with bipolar disorder and has offered help? On the other hand, who shows little interest and makes it clear that helping you is too much of a burden to take on? Who shows little compassion and simply says you need to take care of your "problems"? Trying to change these people is often pointless. The secret is to turn to those who do show an interest in helping you stay stable. The following exercise helps you get clear on who can, can't, or won't become a part of your team.

On the left side, list the people in your daily life. After looking over your list, decide whom you will ask for help and write their names on the right.

People in Your Daily Life	**People You Will Ask for Help**
_____	_____
_____	_____
_____	_____
_____	_____
_____	_____
_____	_____
_____	_____
_____	_____
_____	_____
_____	_____

This list can help you figure out which people don't have the ability or willingness to help you. If you continually ask for help from someone and are continually disappointed, you need to turn to others for help instead of knocking on doors that don't open. This can be difficult if the person is your partner, parent, or best friend, but not everyone is ready to help someone who is ill. Many people have their own issues, and taking on yours might not be something they can do. This doesn't mean that they don't love you or that you stop loving them. It just means that you accept them for who they are and go get help else-where. If their behavior is truly unloving and unkind in other ways, that's a different issue; you may need to limit your contact with this person. But if it's only a problem when you need help for your illness, then turn to someone on your list who is equipped to help you.

■ *For Family and Friends*

Did you know that it's completely normal and fine if you don't want to be one of the people your loved one asks for help? This is the time to be honest. As a friend, maybe you want to be the person who enjoys time with your friend instead of always helping him or her get better. Or perhaps you do want to play a more active role in treatment. As a partner, parent, sibling, grandparent, or other relative, maybe helping someone with such a serious illness is not exactly how you want to live your life. Or maybe you simply don't have the time or energy considering what you are experiencing in your own life. Not everyone is cut out for caretaking. You need to let your loved one know what you can and are willing to do. You have a life and you have the right to be true to yourself. The main idea is to keep your loved one informed instead of just walking away without an explanation. Working on this chapter together is a good way to open the topic and become clear on both sides about what is possible and what isn't. What matters is that you don't feel forced to play a role that makes you resentful or frustrated.

TEACHING YOUR FAMILY AND FRIENDS EXACTLY WHAT THEY CAN DO TO HELP

Now that you're becoming clearer on what you need from your friends and family members and who may be willing to help, you can get more specific and teach them exactly what they can do when you're sick. The following section will help you decide the best ways that the people in your life can help you recognize and hopefully prevent your major bipolar disorder symptoms. Under each major symptom listed below, read the example and then write your ideas on how people can help you when you're ill. You can then show this to the people you've added to your health care team. You will want to do this exercise with all of your major symptoms from this book's introduction. The first example, depression, can serve as a model for how to do this exercise; you can write your own information after the examples.

Example: *Depression.* Here's what works for depression:

- Taking me for a walk or going out with me.
- Asking me if I'm depressed instead of asking me how I am in general.
- Using the tips in this book to help me get stable.
- Knowing the symptoms of depression so that you aren't frustrated and angry when I'm unmotivated, unresponsive, crying, or needy.
- Reminding me that bipolar disorder is an illness and that it has to be treated first.
- Helping me find and eliminate the depression triggers.

_____

_____

_____

_____

_____

■ *For Family and Friends*

You can also do this exercise. Write what you think will help your loved one get better, and then compare your ideas with him or her. You may be amazed at how different your lists are. What you think is effective may sometimes make a mood swing much worse. This is one topic that must be discussed with your loved one. Miscommunication over what actually helps each individual get better is one of the ways you feel frustrated and left out of your loved one's treatment plan.

Example: Here's what doesn't work for depression:

- Telling me that my life is great and there's no reason for me to be so unhappy.
- Getting frustrated and avoiding me because I'm so needy.
- Trying to motivate me to do things without addressing the depression first.
- Telling me to snap out of it.
- Not understanding that it's normal for me to be depressed—it's part of having bipolar disorder and I need help with the illness, not necessarily with my life.

_____

_____

_____

_____

Mania/hypomania. Here's what works for mania and hypomania:

_____

_____

_____

_____

Here's what doesn't work for mania and hypomania:

_____

_____

_____

_____

Anger/irritation. Here's what works for anger/irritation:

_____

_____

_____

_____

_____

Here's what doesn't work for anger/irritation:

_____

_____

_____

_____

_____

Anxiety. Here's what works for anxiety:

_____

_____

_____

_____

_____

Here's what doesn't work for anxiety:

_____

_____

_____

_____

_____

NEEDINESS

One of the main problems with how bipolar disorder affects your relationships is that the illness can make you very needy. It really is a complex and frustrating illness, and you may reach out blindly to whoever is in your life, expecting them to understand what you need and why you need so much, so often. This can be confusing and upsetting for your friends and family members (even those who do want to help) and may cause them to turn away from you. One solution is to have a sort of chain of command you go through before you turn to the same person too many times.

Look over the following chain of command for asking for help. You can add your ideas at the end of the list.

1. I try to help myself first by looking at my lifestyle and deciding on any changes I can make in order to feel better. I use the tips in this book, including changes in diet, exercise, medications, and supplements.
2. I turn to professionals. They're used to my mood swings.
3. I turn to people who understand my needs and are not overwhelmed when I'm sick.
4. I tell the people in my life that I'm ill, and if they offer help, I take it. If not, I look elsewhere.
5. I join professional groups that provide support and kindness when I'm sick. These groups don't have to be related to bipolar disorder.
6. I don't exclusively call one person (such as my mother, father, or best friend) and cry on the phone to them every night. I spread out my needs.
7. I accept that being needy is a sign that I'm depressed, and I have to treat the depression first if I want to end the neediness.
8. I try to get help from friends and family when I really need it instead of just turning to people without thinking of how it will affect them.
9. I accept that my partner may need a break from taking care of me and that I must turn to others instead of burdening one person with all my needs.
10. _____
11. _____
12. _____

> ### ■ *For Family and Friends*
>
> As a family member or friend, where do you want to fit in on this chain of command? Be very clear and let your loved one know what you can and can't handle.

Romantic Relationships

When you're in a relationship with someone and you're sick, it's easy to overburden that person with your neediness. The authors have written a book for the partners of people with bipolar disorder called *Loving Someone with Bipolar Disorder: Understanding and Helping Your Partner* (New Harbinger, 2004). If you're currently in a relationship, you may want to suggest this book to your partner for ideas on how he or she can help you find stability while still maintaining personal health and happiness.

Other Sources for Support

There are many sources you can explore for support outside your friends and family members. One good way to add more people to your life is to join a group of people who share the same hobbies and interests. Do you like crafts? Working on cars? Going to movies? Public speaking? When you join a group of like-minded people, it's possible to have an immediate bond, and these people are often more open to helping you when you need it—you already have a connection. Doing what you love with supportive people is also a great way to increase the brain chemicals you need to maintain a stable mood. Finding a group where you feel comfortable and can do what you love is a good way to find support.

Support Groups

A support group for people with bipolar disorder can be an excellent source of support if the group offers suggestions for healing rather than simply focusing on talking and airing troubles. It can be quite stressful to attend a meeting where everyone is sick and unsure of how to get help. A monitored group is a very good idea. Ask your doctor for resources on how to find these groups. The appendix has suggestions on where to look for support as well.

Unexpected Sources

Sometimes it's the people you don't know well who can help you manage this illness successfully. Is there a kind person at work who shows you special attention? Is there someone you rarely talk to but who has shown an interest in being your friend? Ask that person out for coffee, ask about his or her life, and then talk about yours.

The Internet

Web pages and discussion groups can be a source of support when you're feeling sick. Try to find Web pages and groups that offer a positive and supportive environment for treating the illness. It can be hard to only read about people who are sick and desperate. This can be overwhelming if you're already sick. Look for pages that offer optimistic stories and helpful suggestions on how to get well. Choose your sites and discussion groups carefully. It really does no good to chat over and over again about how sick you are. There are Web page suggestions in the appendix.

Gathering Your Resources

Asking for help isn't always easy. When you're sick, bipolar disorder can make you feel that you have nowhere to go for support. It helps to have a list of people and groups you can turn to when you start to feel as though you're completely alone. Remember, feeling alone and hopeless is a symptom of depression—just as feeling you don't need any help at all is a symptom of mania. The most important thing is to treat bipolar disorder first instead of dwelling on how little help you have in your life. Turn to people and ask for help from those who do have the time for you and then go on from there. Turn to groups and to the Internet when you need support. Constantly remind yourself that this is an illness, not a personal problem. Spread out your needs. The more you teach your friends and family members about the illness, the easier it can be to treat the mood swings. Friends and family are an important part of your health care team. The more educated they are on what this illness does and how they can help you, the more supportive they can be.

Your Toolbox

Knowledge about bipolar disorder.

A correct diagnosis.

A list of your major symptoms.

Medication knowledge.

Help with side effects.

A regular sleep schedule.

A bipolar-friendly diet.

A daily walk.

Regular and appropriate bright light exposure.

A clear picture of your work history.

A clear picture of your current financial position.

A list of your bipolar disorder triggers.

Tips to modify and stop the triggers.

The ability to recognize the bipolar conversation.

A list of leading comments and actions.

The ability to respond instead of reacting to your own bipolar disorder language.

A supportive health care team.

Well-planned appointments.

Friends and family members who can help.

Outside sources of support.

CHAPTER 8

HOSPITALS

Staying in the hospital is a normal part of bipolar disorder for many people. Hospital stays can be extremely traumatic and scary for you and your family and friends, but they are normal. The hospital is a place you go to get stable enough to return to the real world and get on with your life. Unfortunately, many people see hospital visits as something shameful. But the reality is that they are often a lifesaving necessity when a mood swing is too strong for you to take care of at home. The hospital is a safe haven when you are suicidal or so manic that you can no longer function. Seeing hospitalization this way may help you accept the hospital stays you have had in the past. It makes sense that if you are ashamed of your hospital stay, it will be harder for you to ask for help from the people in

■ *For Family and Friends*

For many family members and friends, a trip to the hospital with a loved one is one of the most traumatic experiences they will ever know. The person they love is often gone, and another person seems to be there instead. You wonder if the person you know will ever come back. Will your loved one be this sick forever? Will he or she die? These are all normal questions. The fear you feel is very normal as well. It does end eventually, and the person often gets back to normal, but it takes time and a lot of patience on your part. The more you are able to take care of yourself in this situation and keep on with your life, the more help you can be when your loved one comes home.

your life. This chapter will help you with the shame, embarrassment, and often anger that you feel after a hospital stay so that you can look to others for help in dealing with it.

The chapter covers tips on returning home from the hospital; how to talk to friends, family members, and co-workers about a trip to the hospital; recognizing when you need to go to the hospital; and suggestions on how to prevent hospital visits in the future. One goal of this chapter is to remove the stigma from hospital visits so that you can see the hospital as a place of healing instead of a place of shame. Also, because some people with Bipolar II never experience a hospital visit, this chapter can provide an insight into what happens when someone does need to go to the hospital.

WHEN YOU GET HOME

Hospital visits work for a reason. They offer a low-stimulation environment where a person can focus on healing without having to deal with the outside world. This can't last forever, but a large part of it can be created at home when you come out of the hospital, helping you to maintain stability once you're out of the controlled environment and have to get back to your daily life. The first step is to examine how hospitals help people with bipolar disorder get better:

- Calm, regulated environment.
- Lack of stimulation.
- Almost everything is white.
- Contact with outside people is limited.
- Regular meals.
- Medications are taken care of by someone else.
- Plenty of time for regulated sleep.
- People to help you when you need help.
- Close contact with your doctor and nurses.

Coming out of this controlled environment and going back to your normal life can be quite a shock. You may find that you start to get sick again once you get home. The stress can be enormous, but it's normal when just getting out of the hospital. Taking measures to re-create the hospital environment at home can really make a difference in acclimating back to your regular life. It's also a good idea to re-create some of the hospital environment as a regular part of your home life—this can promote stability and help you stay healthy.

Amanda's Story

Age 25

When my brother got sick, no one knew how to help *me*. My family was in an-other city and his friends were too young to really understand what was going on. I felt completely alone. I didn't know what to say to him when I went to the psych ward. I kept thinking, he's a surfer! He's in college! He likes to drink and hang out with guys. I would go see him in the hospital and he was so skinny and it looked like he hadn't had a bath or brushed his teeth in a month. I couldn't even talk to him without his asking me strange questions like, "Where's the Big Man?" Who in the world was the Big Man? It really scared me. Was the Big Man someone who caused this? Did he do something to end up in the hospital like this? I heard other patients screaming about how they were Jesus and I saw some being held down by four or five nurses because they were so strong. I would go home at night and cry and get really scared. My family finally came and I felt at least like we could be scared together. He finally started to get better after a few months. He was given phone privileges and would call me and say, "Are you still alive? Are you dead?" This really upset me at first. Did someone tell him that? How could he come up with this stuff on his own? We hardly had any deep conversations before he got sick. He was only nineteen. I'm not sure why my parents were not really there. They loved him, but they flew in and flew out so quickly. We were never really a close family. I now think they felt impotent, so they did nothing. After he got out, he stayed with me. We talked about the hospital a lot. I thought he was taking too long to get better especially as he was living with me for free, but now I know that's completely normal. His friends came around and joked with him about how he "went crazy." I think this was very healthy for him. We still live together and his friends still come over. They are there and I'm there and we can work together to make sure he takes the meds and doesn't stay out all night drinking beer anymore. He actually studies. We all look for the signs that he's getting sick again, but not too obviously. He knows we care about him.

In the spaces provided below, list specific ways you can re-create the hospital environment at home:

Sleep: _____

Food: _____

Medications: _____

Asking for help: _____

Limiting stimulation: _____

Many people feel strong emotions after a hospital visit. Whether it's anger at being put in restraints, shame at having tried to kill yourself, or the belief that you were locked up against your will, the emotions can be intense, and they need to be addressed so that you can move forward into managing this illness instead of fighting it. Use the following section to help you work through the emotions you may feel because of a hospital stay.

HOW YOU FEEL ABOUT YOUR HOSPITAL VISIT

You may have been in the hospital years ago, or it may be a recent experience. The question is how you view that hospital visit today. Are you still filled with anger or shame about your stay? Maybe someone you love had to commit you against your will and you're unsure of what to do with your feelings of anger and hurt. Or maybe you feel ashamed at

■ *For Family and Friends*

Family members or friends are often the people who take care of a person when he or she leaves the hospital. If you have any control over the environment when your loved one comes home, try to re-create the hospital environment as best you can. Remove all disturbing photos, books, and videos. Remove any art, writing, or destruction that your loved one may have done when first sick. Keep the bedroom clean and uncluttered. Have space for your loved one to rest and get used to being home again.

having to go to the hospital for help. Maybe you think you should have been able to deal with your problems on your own. There is also a chance that your friends and family members made you feel weak for needing so much help. Think about how you want to work on these emotions. You can talk with a therapist, your doctor, a support group, an online chat group, or a trusted friend or family member about these feelings. The goal is to get these emotions out in the open so that they don't hamper your recovery once you're home. You can fill out the following exercise and then take this book with you when you see your doctor, visit a therapist, or talk with a friend.

Put a check next to the emotions you identify with. After you get an idea of your emotional position, you will be better able to discuss your feelings with your family, friends, and health care professionals.

☐ Ashamed.
☐ Scared.
☐ Confused.
☐ Angry.
☐ Helpless.
☐ Worried about the future.
☐ Tired.
☐ Worried about work.
☐ Depressed.
☐ Suicidal.

☐ Worried about money.
☐ Feel like an outcast.
☐ Worried about what others will think.
☐ Don't think I'll ever get back to normal.
☐ Scared I'll have to go back.
☐ Scared I will never work again.
☐ Feel that my life is ruined forever.
☐ Don't think I can discuss things with you.
☐ Feel that people don't understand.
☐ Feel pressured to get back to normal.

■ For Family and Friends

When your loved one comes out of the hospital, don't act as though nothing happened and things are back to normal; ask questions. For most people, a hospital visit remains a part of their lives forever. It can be traumatic and life changing. The more you respect this, the easier the transition back to normal life will be for your loved one. When he or she seems well enough to answer your questions, ask. There is no shame in being so sick that you need to go to the hospital because of bipolar disorder. Don't tiptoe around. Don't be scared to be honest.

COMING TO TERMS WITH WHAT YOU
DID BEFORE YOU WENT TO THE HOSPITAL

You may have done some very unwise things when you were sick. Some people end up in jail, others have affairs, some engage in dangerous behaviors such as wrecking a car or taking an overdose of pills. Others spend thousands of dollars and ruin their family financially. Some people leave their normal life and get on a plane for a trip around the world, while others make detrimental financial decisions that break up families and change their lives forever. It helps if you can face these behaviors head-on, accept that they were part of the illness, try to repair what you can, and then make a decision to use the ideas in this book to make sure that you never get so sick again. The point is not to make light of what might have happened, but rather to acknowledge that this illness makes people do things they would never do if they weren't sick. Try to forgive yourself for what happened, make sincere apologies when you can, and use the tips in this book to make sure it never happens again.

Using the space below, write down your behaviors before you were hospitalized. As you write, remind yourself that you're not the first person with bipolar disorder to make stupid, dangerous, life-changing mistakes when you were sick. Go easy on yourself. Face the reality, but remind yourself that the reality is that you have an illness that, if untreated, often leads to this kind of behavior. After each problem you list, write what you're going to do to make sure it never happens again. An example is provided.

Problem: Reached the limit on all of my credit cards. I'm now over twenty thousand dollars in debt and it only took two months. I feel such shame and worry over what I did when I was manic. When I got out of the hospital, the reality hit me so hard that I got depressed. How am I going to get my life back?

Solutions: Take my medications so that mania never takes over my life again. Get financial help to pay off the debt. Talk with creditors, return what I can, ask for help, and explain in very clear terms that it was an illness that made me spend this way. Set up checks and balances so this never happens again. Talk with others who have similar problems so that I can see it's not me, but an illness.

Problem: _____

_____

_____

_____

_____

Solutions: _____

_____

_____

_____

_____

Retracing Your Path to the Hospital

Hospital visits often seem to come out of the blue. Friends and family will say, "He was so normal one day, and then he just snapped and had to go to the hospital for three weeks." Or, "She seemed fine, and then we found her with a bottle of pills and some wine, and we had to rush her to the hospital." This is not actually a realistic picture of what leads up to a hospital visit. *Hospital visits never come out of a void.* Behavior that leads to hospitalization is often present weeks and even months before the final decision is made to go to the

■ *For Family and Friends*

How did your loved one's pre-hospital behavior affect your life? What do you need to do to get over your resentment and frustration if he used your money, went to jail and you had to bail him out, tried to kill himself in your home, had sex with someone you know, acted crazy in public, lost his job, or yelled at you and said his problems were all your fault? What if she scared you or a younger sibling? What if she refused hospitalization and you had to have her committed? All of this must be talked about in a rational and calm manner when your loved one is well enough to talk. If you ignore these issues, they will only get bigger and bigger and your resentment will grow exponentially even though you rationally know that the behavior was caused by an illness.

hospital. There are always signs. It's natural that someone who has not been diagnosed with bipolar disorder would have no idea what signs to look for, but now that you have a diagnosis, you can learn your own signs in order to prevent future hospital visits.

If you were in the hospital, think of your behaviors in the weeks before you were admitted. Think of your sleep, eating, socializing, work, money, and relationship choices. What did others notice? Did anyone try to help you? Write all of this down below. You will then use this information to look for signs in the future that you may be heading for a hospital visit. You can write ideas in the solutions section on what you can do as soon as you see the signs that you're getting sick enough to need the hospital. An example is provided.

Pre-hospital symptoms: Felt down when I woke up. Wondered why my life was so pointless. Started to think about dying. The feelings were so real, I honestly thought my life was worthless. When my family said something, I just said I was going through some changes and that they should leave me alone. I had no idea what was happening. I stopped working, and soon couldn't even answer the phone. I couldn't be with people or smile or have fun. Soon I was consumed with the idea that I wanted to die, and I tried to kill myself.

Solutions: I can make a list of what I was thinking and feeling, and show it to the people in my life so that they know what to look for. I can take my medications and have regular doctor's appointments as a check-in. I can now know that the first little signs, such as thinking that life is pointless, mean I need immediate help; I can't wait until I actually try to kill myself. I have to get help way before then.

Your pre-hospital symptoms: _____

_____

_____

_____

Your solutions: _____

_____

For Family and Friends

As a family member or friend, you will need to be prepared for a hospital visit, especially if your loved one has been in the hospital in the past. What hospital will you go to? What paperwork will you need? Do you know what medications your loved one is taking? Who will you have to talk to to get him or her admitted? It really helps to think ahead. Going to the hospital can be so stressful that you often forget what you need to do.

If your family member does go to the hospital, make your own list of the signs you saw before he went. Then compare it with his or her own list. What can you do together to prevent another visit? What can you write down and both sign that says, *As soon as I see this set of symptoms, we will go to the doctor together and get help before a hospital visit is needed*? Hospital visits can be prevented, and because family members and friends are often the first people to see the signs that a mood swing is starting, you need to have a plan for what to do the minute you see these signs.

_____

_____

_____

Your Physical Body Needs Recovery, Too

Your body goes through extreme chemical changes when you have a serious bipolar disorder episode. The body's regulatory system is off; normal self-maintenance is often impossible when you're sick. When you combine this with the new medications you will take after you're diagnosed, the impact on your physical body can be intense. You need time to recover physically if you were in the hospital for an episode. This is a time when it's especially important to use the tips in chapter 2 on sleep, diet, exercise, and light. Go easy on yourself and give yourself time to mentally and physically heal from a hospital stay.

■ *For Family and Friends*

One of the biggest mistakes that family members and friends make is to think that recovery from a hospital stay should be quick. The facts are these: It can take people a year or more to recover from a serious hospital stay. Their minds and bodies have been through a terrifically stressful experience. Their physical bodies are exhausted and they need time. If you plan for a year of recovery, you can be more understanding when your loved one doesn't get better in your time frame.

TALKING ABOUT THE HOSPITAL EXPERIENCE

Mental illness is still a taboo topic for many people. Psychiatric wards in hospitals are unmarked. The wards are often locked and security is high. This can affect the way you view your hospital stay and the people who came to see you. It's not like you went to a colorful ward with fellow patients there for minor surgery or to have a baby. You were around some very ill and, often at first, very scary people. Then after you were there for a while, you realized that you were surrounded by people like yourself who needed help for mental illness. There was no reason to be embarrassed or ashamed at being in the hospital. Then you had to go home and talk about your experience, often to people who had no way of understanding what you went through. Or, if you're like many people, you wanted to go home and forget about your experience, but people wanted to know what happened. The goal of this section is to help you find the words to explain why you were in the hospital.

It may help if you first write down what you want to say. Sometimes it's useful to create a script you can use when you're faced with difficult questions from friends, family, and co-workers. Read the following example and then write one of your own.

As you may know, I was just in the hospital. I have an illness called bipolar disorder. Many people with bipolar disorder have to go into the hospital, especially when they are first diagnosed. I know that my behavior seemed bizarre to you, but this is why I needed help. The illness makes me do a lot of strange and unexplainable things. I had to go to the hospital to get my brain chemistry regulated so that I could get back to my normal life. I can learn to manage this illness, but sometimes I need the help of a hospital setting. It's very calm there, and I can just focus on getting better. It's a bit hard when I get out, and I could use your help and understanding. If you have any questions about bipolar disorder, I can help answer them.

Write your script here:

_____

_____

_____

_____

_____

_____

_____

_____

_____

_____

Explaining What Happened and Why You Acted as You Did

How can you explain a suicide attempt? What if you were violent when you were manic and psychotic? What if you hurt someone emotionally or scared your kids? You may wonder how people with bipolar disorder get through this shame and pain. Often it's by being

■ *For Family and Friends*

You can write a script for those times when someone asks why your loved one acted so oddly and had to go to the hospital. Don't be ashamed of your loved one and his or her behavior. Bipolar disorder is an illness. You wouldn't be ashamed to talk about a loved one's ordeal in the hospital for cancer, right?

honest, by keeping a dialogue open with the people in your life, and by accepting that there may be things you can't repair; you have to let them go. It helps if you're understanding of yourself and don't keep beating yourself up for what you did when you were sick. As said many times in this book, bad, strange, scary, and unimaginable behaviors can happen when you're in a serious episode. The problem is that there will be times when you will have to explain these behaviors to others. Some people will listen and understand, and some won't. You then have to move on and use your comprehensive treatment plan to make sure the behaviors rarely happen again. It's often like starting over. And starting over can be very scary, but it can be done. It's better than repeating the mistakes of the past again and again.

What You Want to Say

Using the tips you have learned in this book, write down what you want to say to someone in your life whom you may have hurt or scared by your behavior before you went to the hospital. Be honest. Remind yourself and them that it's an illness and that you're now on medications and getting help in managing the illness as a whole. The person you're talking to may have been very traumatized by your hospital stay, so be thoughtful and gentle as you talk.

What you want to say to the people you've hurt or scared:

_____

_____

_____

_____

_____

_____

_____

_____

_____

HOW TO PREVENT ANOTHER TRIP TO THE HOSPITAL

You *can* prevent a return trip to the hospital. It will take a lot of teamwork, and you will need to use the suggestions in this book as well as the help from your health care providers, but it can be done. The following list offers some tips on how to prevent a trip to the hospital. Add your own ideas, and ask your friends and family members for their thoughts as well:

- Know the first symptoms of a mood swing so that you can get immediate help.
- Have a good relationship with your doctor and other health care professionals so that they can monitor your mood swings.
- Chart your mood swings daily when you're first diagnosed, to see your patterns. Appendix C has a chart you can use.
- Ask others to look for signs and talk with you openly if they think you're getting sick.
- Monitor your spending carefully. When spending gets out of control, it's often a sign that bipolar disorder needs to be treated immediately.
- Watch your thoughts carefully. Suicidal thoughts, whether passive or active, are always a sign that you need help. Don't let these thoughts go too far.
- Make sure that your medications are working and that you're taking them regularly.
- Beware of alcohol and drug use. An increase in these behaviors is often a sign that you're getting sick.

Write your ideas here on how you can prevent hospital visits:

_____

_____

_____

_____

_____

Terrence's Story

Age 31

On my twenty-first birthday, after a trip to Europe, I went into such a bad manic episode I stayed in a state hospital for almost six months. I'm sure my family wanted me to come home, but they kept telling me it was better if I stayed. Of course I now know they were right, but at the time I wanted to kill them. How could they let the nurses treat me like this? They held me down! They put straps on my arms! I remember thinking, *What in the hell are they doing? Who told them to do this? Where are my rights?* And yet, I must have only thought this after I was better. My family and friends told me stories I couldn't believe. That I wrapped a towel around my head and said I was an Arab prince or that I heard gunshots all day and would jump at any sound. I couldn't put on my own clothes and had no idea how to brush my own teeth. Before I lost the ability to write, I made a detailed list of all I had to do to take a shower: take off shoes, remove pants, underwear, et cetera. I was reduced to being a child. When I got home I was filled with such rage. I wanted to get back at people for letting this happen to me. And when I said this, my father said, "What were we supposed to do? You were so manic you couldn't say one coherent sentence. You talked about saving people's lives and helping your sister learn to parallel park better and that you had discovered the cure for cancer by using a new strain of cancer cells." I didn't remember much of that. I do remember trying to write a check and I couldn't do it, and at one point I was in a grocery store talking to all of the customers about fruit. Now it's like a dream. What I'm slowly realizing is that it was *not* a dream for my family. It was a solid nightmare. I can talk about it more rationally now. I never went back to the hospital.

Recognizing the Signs That You Need Immediate Help

It's very possible that your illness will someday grow too strong again, and you will have to return to the hospital. One way to make this easier is to make sure you know the signs that you need help before you make life-altering decisions. If you can create a list of the signs that you need immediate help and show this to your friends, family members, and health care team, they can help you get medical attention immediately instead of the mood swing going so far that you need to be committed against your will. Read over the following examples and add your symptoms to the end of the list.

Signs That You Need Immediate Help

- Active suicidal thoughts that don't respond to medications.
- Mania or depression that can no longer be treated at home.
- Dangerous behavior.
- An inability to do anything, including getting out of bed, eating, working, or having a normal conversation.
- Talk of dying.
- Canceling doctor's appointments even when it's obvious that you need them.
- Reverting to old behaviors.
- Stopping all medications and saying you're cured when it's obvious to others that you're still sick.
- Crying that won't stop.

_____

_____

_____

_____

_____

Hospital Visits

Even though prevention can deter hospital visits, the illness is simply too strong sometimes and you will need the safety of a hospital. This is nothing to be ashamed of.

For many people, it can take a year (yes, a year) or more to recover from a stay in the hospital. Bipolar disorder is a serious illness, both mentally and physically. Your mind and body need time to recover, and you need time to adjust to your medications and the reality of having a lifelong mental illness. This takes time. It's important that you give yourself time to heal. It's also very important that you ask for help, because getting better on your own can be quite difficult. Even though hospital visits are often a normal part of having bipolar disorder, they can still be traumatic. The more you can work on accepting hospitals as a normal part of the illness for many people, the easier it can be for you to re-cover, ask for help, and go on with your life. As with all parts of bipolar disorder, preven-tion is the key. The 4-Step Treatment Plan helps you find the stability needed to stay well enough so that you hopefully won't need another hospital visit in the future.

Your Toolbox

Knowledge about bipolar disorder.

A correct diagnosis.

A list of your major symptoms.

Medication knowledge.

Help with side effects.

A regular sleep schedule.

A bipolar-friendly diet.

A daily walk.

Regular and appropriate bright light exposure.

A clear picture of your work history.

A clear picture of your current financial position.

A list of your bipolar disorder triggers.

Tips to modify and stop the triggers.

The ability to recognize the bipolar conversation.

A list of leading comments and actions.

The ability to respond instead of reacting to your own bipolar disorder language.

A supportive health care team.

Well-planned appointments.

Friends and family members who can help.

Outside sources of support.

A plan to prevent hospital visits.

CHAPTER 9

INSURANCE AND PAPERWORK

Managing an illness is often a difficult and time-consuming project. It can become even more difficult if you think of all of the paperwork you will need to fill out and organize regarding bipolar disorder. When you add this to managing insurance or finding help if you don't have insurance, the logistics of managing this illness can be overwhelming. It's especially difficult if you're sick right now or have just come out of the hospital.

One goal of this chapter is to help you create a filing system you can use to keep track of all of the paperwork, so that it's not overwhelming or stressful. You'll learn how to keep track of what you will need to fill out and have with you during bipolar-disorder-related appointments, as well as how to organize the paperwork you already have for easy access. The last part of the chapter covers insurance. The first insurance section will help you manage the insurance paperwork you may already have, while the second part will offer suggestions on how to get help if you currently don't have insurance.

TIPS FOR DEALING WITH PAPERWORK WHEN YOU'RE SICK

Paperwork can feel completely overwhelming when you're sick. The irony is that in order to get help and financial assistance, you have to fill out this paperwork, but the reason you need help and assistance is that you're too sick to do anything, much less the paperwork. It's totally normal if you don't feel well enough to complete paperwork when you're having mood swings, but the reality is that the bills and forms do not go away just because you're sick. Once you have your papers organized, you will at least know what needs to be done, and it will no longer be a large paper monster following you around and making you feel guilty.

Still, dealing with *all* the paperwork generated by bipolar disorder may simply be impossible for you right now. Or maybe the stress of not having insurance and trying to find low-cost health care is just too much for you to handle. If this is the case, you will have to ask for help. Do you have a social worker who can help you get organized? Or a friend who can look at all the papers and help you to create the filing system described below? Whom can you ask today for help? Is there a support group where you can all bring your paperwork and get it organized together? You may have to get creative here and think outside the box. But don't let the papers just sit in a pile creating late notices and more trouble for you in the future. That will only cause more illness. Getting organized can be such a relief and can give you more space to use the suggestions in this book to get better.

CREATING A BIPOLAR DISORDER FILING SYSTEM

Considering that bipolar disorder is an illness that needs to be managed daily, it helps if you have a filing system dedicated to management. You can then take this system with you to all of your health care appointments, avoiding the need to constantly look for paperwork and information when you're sick or stressed. It makes a big difference to have everything in one place, especially if you have a lot of appointments related to bipolar disorder.

The following system uses a single accordion file that you can buy at any office-supply store. Look for a file that has pockets large enough to hold this book and an appointment

■ *For Family and Friends*

Just as with the bipolar conversation, insurance and paperwork is an area where you can make a significant difference when your loved one is ill. It may be hard for you to imagine, but a task as simple as filling out a form is often too overwhelming for someone in a bipolar disorder mood swing. Just sitting with your loved one and doing the writing can relieve the stress many people feel when confronted with a pile of questionnaires, insurance forms, and drug information.

book. Make sure that the file closes easily and that the sections are large enough to hold separate manila folders. The accordion file should be large enough to hold all your paperwork, but small enough to carry with you. Label each section with the following headings:

Appointment Book
Bills
Disability/Assistance
Insurance
Medications
Bipolar Disorder Information
Hospital
To Do

You can then use labeled manila folders in each section to more effectively file your paperwork. For example, under INSURANCE, you can have one manila folder for all

Ethan's Story

Age 49

Creating the bipolar file was one of the smartest things I did when I first got diagnosed. It's like every time I go to the doctor, they hand me more stuff. A copy of my bill, insurance information, and these little pamphlets on all of the drugs I'm taking. It's really too much to read at once. It *does* help to file it immediately. I used to worry so much about where my bills were and when they were due. When I'm too sick to file, which means the depression is so bad I can't even open the file box, it seems so overwhelming, I hand everything to my friend and she files it for me. I didn't have any insurance for years and then my state offered a plan that I finally qualified for. It is not cheap, so I ask family and friends for help. They know where to send the money and they know it's one way they can help me stay stable. I also ask them to help me manage the insurance paperwork. That is always difficult. It's great to have one place for all of my bipolar stuff. I can just pick up one file and take it with me to the doctor.

receipts and co-pays, one for policies, and one for contact information. Under the BILLS heading, you can have a separate folder for bills yet to pay, and one for paid bills. You may have three or more folders within each section. You can keep your appointment book in the file, as well as this book. Every time you receive new paperwork or have a new appointment, all the information can go directly in your filing system with limited stress. You can then take the whole accordion file to your appointments and know that you have everything you need. You can also make copies of the charts in appendix C and file them in your system. And finally, it's not a bad idea to put this book in your file. It may help to reread some of the tips in the book before your appointment.

HOSPITAL PAPERWORK

If you were in the hospital and now have bills to pay, it's important that you get all the paperwork in one place. You can then talk with the hospital or your insurance company to find out exactly what you owe and when it needs to be paid. Your bipolar disorder filing system can help you to get all this paperwork in one place. It's also important that you keep track of your hospital visits. There is a chart in appendix C that can help you with this process. This is also a good record for your family to have if they must help you check into the hospital. If you're not sure of the dates, ask for a copy of any information you need from your doctor. Getting the information on paper may seem like a lot of work at first, but having it all in one place can really make a difference if you need to apply for assistance or tell a new health care professional your history.

INSURANCE

Many people with insurance are not fully aware of what they're actually charged for services and how much their policy covers in case of an emergency or hospitalization. Once a crisis happens, it's often scary to see how limited the coverage is or how much the deductible or co-payment can be in certain situations. It's important that you're fully aware of the coverage and cost of your insurance policy. See if you can answer the following:

- What exactly does my policy cover?
- Do I have a group or individual policy?
- Do I have co-pays or deductibles?
- When does the policy renew?
- If my policy is through my work, how much do I pay each month out of my paycheck?
- What is the coverage for lab tests or X-rays?
- Does the policy cover emergency room visits?
- What is the coverage for hospital stays?
- What complementary treatments does my policy cover?
- What is the coverage for medications? Do I have different co-pays depending on the type of medication I need?
- Does my insurance have a yearly limit? How do I know when I reach this limit?

Don't worry if you can't answer all of these questions. You may have to call your insurance company or ask for help from the human resource department where you work. It may take a bit of research and time at first to find the answers to these questions, but it's worth having this information all in one place. Appendix C has charts you can fill out that will help you organize it. Knowing this information and adding it to your file system can reduce stress and can help your friends and family find what they need if you become too sick to help yourself.

Appendix C

Appendix C has a place for you to chart your insurance information. You can fill out the forms and then put them in your file to take with you to your appointments for easy access to the information.

Tips for Tracking Your Insurance Claims

Once you have more information on your actual policy, you will need to track your insurance claims carefully. The following tips can help you with this process:

- Carry your accordion file with you to every doctor's visit.
- Use the co-pay sheet in appendix C to record any co-pays or deductibles.
- Ask for a copy of the bill each time you visit a doctor. This prevents later surprises. You can then put this bill directly into the file.
- Get a receipt for any co-pay or deductible and put it in the insurance section of your accordion file immediately.
- Make sure that your doctor is sending in the claim to your insurance company.
- When you get your statement, make sure that everything is in order.
- If you find a problem, call your insurance company immediately and then note the results of the call in your accordion file.

Understanding your insurance policy is all about stress reduction. Sometimes this paperwork can feel impossible to deal with when you're sick, so the more you have in order before you get sick, the easier it will be to find the information when you need help. It also helps if your family knows what is covered and where they can find your insurance information in case they have to help you go to the hospital. It's a good idea to show them the system you set up with your accordion file so that they know where to go for information.

No Insurance? What Are Your Options?

Not having insurance is a large problem for many people with bipolar disorder. The illness is hard enough to deal with without having to worry about getting the health care

---

If You Don't Have Insurance

You can apply for individual insurance and see what happens. You may be surprised and get accepted; if not, the insurance company is obligated to send you information on insurance alternatives. This is invaluable. There are also many sites on the Internet where you can apply for insurance online. It's easy, and it will at least let you see your options if you do get rejected.

---

you need, but the reality is that many people don't have insurance, either because they can't work, their work doesn't offer insurance, or they don't have the money to pay the premiums. For some people, the bipolar disorder diagnosis prevents them from getting individual insurance coverage. It can really be a vicious cycle if you're not already protected by insurance when you're first diagnosed. If you don't have insurance right now, the following list offers some suggestions on the next steps you can take.

- Contact local mental health advocacy groups to ask for help with your options. Resources are provided in appendix A.
- Call an insurance agent and ask for help. You may have more options than you think.
- Know your county system and what is available to you. Ask the following questions of your doctor and any other member of your health care team:

  Where should I go and whom should I see to find out what services are available to me?

  Where do I go if I don't have enough money for medications?

  What are my options if I don't have insurance?

  I need to find an advocate to help me find alternatives to insurance. Do you have any suggestions?

  Where can I go for information on low-cost and sliding-scale-fee help with doctor's visits and medications?

  Where can I find a therapist who charges on a sliding scale?

- You can also go to an online chat group and ask for suggestions from people who live in your area.

■ *For Family and Friends*

It's often very difficult to watch someone you love go through insurance problems when they're diagnosed with bipolar disorder. The illness is hard enough without having to worry about paying for competent treatment. One way you can help, if it's financially feasible, is to pool people together to pay for an insurance policy. This is one of the greatest gifts you can give to a person with bipolar disorder—it provides stability.

■ Contact a discount medical services company. These companies offer discount medical services where you can pay a fee per month and then receive discounted services and medications from certain providers. Once you sign up for this service, you will receive a list of accepted providers. You can then call them to see what discount they offer. Discounts may be as little as 20 percent, so this service is only worth the monthly fee if you spend more than the fee each month. If you search the Internet under "insurance alternatives," you can find more information on these services. They're at least an option if you are unable to get insurance.
■ Explore Medicaid and Medicare.
■ Don't lose hope. There is an option out there for you. What matters is that you get your medications and the help you need. If you can't do this yourself, then ask someone to help you. It may be hard to get things set up, but once they are in place you will have more time to work on the suggestions in this book. Remember that nothing is forever. Once your illness is better managed, there is a good chance that you can go back to work and get insurance from your employer.

DON'T PUT OFF THE PAPERWORK

One of the biggest mistakes people make when they're ill is letting things slide until they feel well enough to take care of them. This simply won't work if you have payment due dates, appointments, and other paperwork obligations. As hard as it may be right now, you have to think of the future and remind yourself that getting a letter from a bill collector can cause more stress than sitting down and getting your papers organized as soon as possible. What step can you take right now to get started?

Once you have a system in place for managing your paperwork, the overwhelmed feelings can end, and you can be assured that you have one place for all of your bipolar disorder paperwork needs. If you have insurance, then you will be more aware of what the policy covers. If you don't have insurance, a good paperwork system will help you decide the next steps you need to take to find appropriate health care. Give yourself time to create this system and get everything organized, but try to start today. The relief can be worth the effort.

Your Toolbox

Knowledge about bipolar disorder.

A correct diagnosis.

A list of your major symptoms.

Medication knowledge.

Help with side effects.

A regular sleep schedule.

A bipolar-friendly diet.

A daily walk.

Regular and appropriate bright light exposure.

A clear picture of your work history.

A clear picture of your current financial position.

A list of your bipolar disorder triggers.

Tips to modify and stop the triggers.

The ability to recognize the bipolar conversation.

A list of leading comments and actions.

The ability to respond instead of reacting to your own bipolar disorder language.

A supportive health care team.

Well-planned appointments.

Friends and family members who can help.

Outside sources of support.

A plan to prevent hospital visits.

An understanding of your insurance policy.

Well-ordered and up-to-date paperwork in one file.

PUTTING IT ALL TOGETHER
Using the 4-Step Treatment Plan in Daily Life

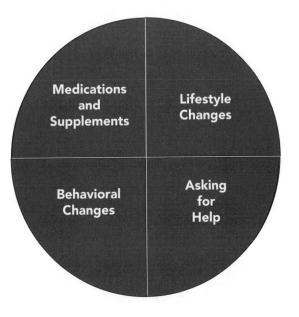

CHAPTER 10

SPECIFIC PLANS
FOR SPECIFIC PROBLEMS

Now that you have learned the tips in the 4-Step Plan regarding medications and supplements, lifestyle changes, behavior changes, and asking for help, you are ready to apply your knowledge of managing the illness to specific bipolar disorder problems. Bipolar disorder can create a variety of issues in your life that can often seem overwhelming—especially if you're newly diagnosed or are having trouble with your medications. Creating a plan for each problem separately can help you manage the illness in small sections and help ease these overwhelming feelings.

This chapter covers ten common bipolar disorder problems and offers tips on how to manage each. The goal is to help you use the tools from earlier chapters to create a management plan for each problem you face. You can then use the plans you create in this chapter for other issues that arise when you get sick.

■ *For Family and Friends*

As a family member or friend, you can fill out this chapter on your own, then compare your ideas with your loved one's. As we've said many times, it's often the people on the outside looking in who can spot behaviors your loved one can't. You can give your loved one a unique perspective on your ideas for treating the illness successfully. And if the person with the illness is not open to your ideas, at least you have more tools to help you take care of yourself.

■ *For Family and Friends*

For some people with bipolar disorder, asking for help is difficult, while others ask for so much help they overwhelm their family members, friends, and health care professionals. This is your chance to write down what you see your loved one do and then talk about more effective strategies for meeting his or her needs. This may take some time simply because people who are ill are often unable to communicate what they need without being overly emotional, or are so numbed or drugged they don't show any emotions at all. But don't give up. The more tactics you and your loved one have for managing the illness, the less stress there will be on your relationship.

THE STEPS

The following exercises will take you through the process of creating a management plan for ten separate problems. There are five steps in each of the following exercises:

1. Symptoms
2. Medications
3. Triggers
4. Asking for help
5. Lifestyle changes I can make

Symptoms

Knowing the initial symptoms of the problems you experience because of bipolar disorder is a great first step to recognizing the problem, and hopefully preventing it from going any farther and affecting your life adversely. As you write down your first symptoms, remind yourself of what you say, do, and think each time the problem starts. Remember to write your leading comments and actions. Try to think of the first indications that the problem is starting and get them on paper so that you can recognize them as reminders to treat bipolar disorder first.

Medications

The medications section is a place for you to examine your current medications. Are you on the right meds? Are they contributing to the problem? Is your dose high enough? Are you taking the medications as prescribed? Do you need different ones? These questions will help you become more aware of how your medications affect your life and how important it is for you to closely monitor and track them, so that you are ready with questions when you see your doctor. Use this section to write your ideas on how you can effectively use medications to help you find answers to the problem.

Triggers

Chapter 4 taught you that there are many situations, people, and events, as well as your own behaviors, that can trigger bipolar disorder symptoms. As you look over the problems listed, think of what might trigger the problem or cause it to get worse. You can then list the top triggers for the problem and start working on modifying or eliminating them.

Asking for Help

It may be hard to ask for help for some of the issues in this chapter. When mania goes too far, for example, asking for help may be almost impossible. The goal of this section is to get you to write down your ideas about where to go for help before you actually need the help. Then, when you notice the first symptoms of a problem, you can go to this section and read your own ideas on how to manage the situation.

Lifestyle Changes I Can Make

Ultimately, even with a serious illness such as bipolar disorder, it's often up to you to make the changes you need to make in order to stay well. This can be very difficult if you have learned many bad habits due to bipolar disorder, but change needs to happen if you want to find stability. When you look over each problem and notice its symptoms and triggers, think about the first small changes you can make to at least start dealing with the issue. It will be easier to make larger and more difficult changes once you see how the small changes can make a difference.

Finding Ideas

You can take ideas from other chapters as well as from your health care team, friends, and family members. This would also be a good chapter to use in a support group or with your therapist. You don't have to fill out this chapter completely. You can add ideas as you work with your health care professionals as well. You can then use this system for treating any other bipolar-disorder-related problems that you want to work on. Each section starts with some suggestions, and then has a space for you to add your own ideas. There is a final entry where you can work on one of your own problems using the ideas in this chapter.

MANIC DISASTERS

Manic disasters, from inappropriate sexual behavior and excessive spending to agitation and making life-changing, spur-of-the-moment decisions, can really wreck your life. The

■ *For Family and Friends*

Family members and friends are often the first to notice signs that mania is starting. For some reason, they rarely say anything until after a lot of damage has been done. Then they get upset with the person for being manic—and yet they saw the signs and could have done something before it was too late. There are many reasons for this. The person you are trying to help may get really mad and push you away. He or she may not listen and will just go on with the behavior because he or she can't help it. This is part of the illness. The *only* way to deal with this is to have a plan in place to deal with mania way before it starts. Read over what your loved one says in this section about mania and talk about it together. Create a plan so you both know the very first signs of mania; write down the plan. Then you can take it out when the symptoms start. This often gets through to the ill person better than your talking or lecturing. Reading something he or she wrote when well is a powerful deterrent to mood swings. And finally, it's totally up to you to protect yourself against manic disasters. This may cause some pain at first, especially if you have a partner with bipolar disorder and you want to separate all your money. Still, it's better than losing everything you have because of one serious manic mood swing.

best way to deal with these manic disasters is to prevent them from ever happening again. Mania is difficult to treat once it goes too far. Because of this, you need to learn the first signs of your mania symptoms, write them down, show them to your friends and family members, and have a plan ready to implement the minute the symptoms start. This section will help you start your plan to prevent manic disasters. You can write your own information after the examples.

Symptoms

- Saying things like, "Can't you just let me have some fun for once?"
- Finally feeling good and wanting to make up for the time I lost when I was depressed.
- Starting to impulsively spend money.
- Needing a lot less sleep and it feels so good!

_____

_____

_____

_____

_____

Medications

- I'm taking a new medication. I will ask my doctor if it can cause mania.
- I missed a few doses of my medication.
- I stopped taking meds because I felt so good.
- Am I taking any medications to prevent mania?

_____

_____

_____

_____

Triggers

- Vacation.
- New job that has been really stressful.
- Business trip to a different time zone.
- Going out more than usual and sleeping a lot less.

_____

_____

_____

_____

_____

Asking for Help

- Call my doctor right now and say I think I'm getting manic.
- Teach the people in my life the first signs that I'm getting manic so that they can help me before it goes too far.
- Set up regular appointments with my doctor to check in even if I feel good.
- Involve my friends and family in helping me prevent mania.

_____

_____

_____

_____

_____

Lifestyle Changes I Can Make

- Make sure I get to bed at the same time every night.
- Stop drinking caffeine at night.
- Accept that I can't go out and party like I want to.
- Say no to extra projects at work.

_____

_____

_____

_____

■ *For Family and Friends*

This is your chance to tell your loved one what you need when he or she asks for help with mania. Do you feel frustrated when he ignores your concerns about mania? Are you frustrated that she doesn't ask for help from the right people and uses drugs, alcohol, or inappropriate friends for support? This is your place to write all of this down. You can use the skills you learned in chapter 5, The Bipolar Conversation, to fill in these sections.

Ben's Story

Age 40

Mania feels really good at first. Spending money feels like being in love. Everything feels like being in love. All the food in restaurants looks amazing. I will look at a menu and it all sounds so good, I can't make a choice. People look great! I can walk up to anyone and say hi and they will talk to me. I *love* to drink. It tastes so good! Sex! Wow! Talking on the phone all night. Getting my work done in half the time. It's all amazing. I guess this is why I ignored the reality of mania for so many years. This amazing stuff doesn't last. Ever. People start to get really annoyed with me. They want to sleep. They look at me like I'm a maniac. Wow, I never thought of the meaning of that word! My love affair with mania ended a few years ago when I left my partner and children and flew to Mexico for a condo deal. I lost a lot of money. My partner was scared and angry, and said this was the last time she would go through this. I ended up drunk in a hotel in Mazatlán with a strange woman. My mood started to go down and I got really scared. I could tell this was the last time I wanted to go through this. I managed to get on a plane and went straight to my doctor. I've been on medication ever since. I *dream* about the mania. I miss the good stuff. But when I think of going off the meds, I remember that hotel room and the alcohol and the woman. My marriage didn't survive all of this, but we have a good relationship now and my kids are in my life. I can work again and I feel things are getting better. I will always long for mania, but I have a system that works now. I won't go back there.

RELATIONSHIP PROBLEMS

Bipolar disorder is really hard on relationships. From neediness to unreliability, paranoia, insensitivity, acting moody, and feeling terribly lonely, bipolar disorder can make you a difficult person to be around. One of the best ways to keep your relationships strong even when you're having mood swings is to learn to recognize the signs that you're getting sick—especially those that may cause problems in your relationships. You can then treat the illness instead of taking out your problems on the people around you.

Symptoms

- Saying things like, "I don't think you really care about me."
- Feeling lonely all the time—or needing too much from others and overwhelming people.

■ *For Family and Friends*

It may be that you personally have problems with your loved one because of bipolar disorder. You probably notice that people with this illness can have more relationship issues than most people. This makes sense when you consider that relationships are quite emotional even when you don't have bipolar disorder. Can you imagine what it's like to have to deal with relationships when your brain tells you things that aren't true? Your help, guidance, and understanding can really make a difference.

If you're friends with someone who has bipolar disorder, you know how difficult it can be to know what mood your friend is in. Maybe, as mentioned before, you have received a paranoid e-mail in which your friend asks what's wrong and why you don't like him or her anymore. Maybe your friend is hot and cold or too needy. It can be very difficult to remain friends with someone who has a lot of mood swings. It may simply be impossible to maintain the friendship if the person refuses medications and doesn't think he or she is sick at all.

■ Pushing people away—or getting irritated really easily.
■ Talking too fast and overwhelming people.

_____

_____

_____

_____

_____

Medications

■ Check to see if my medication dose is correct.
■ Make sure I'm being treated for depression correctly.
■ Is there a medication that can help with these feelings?
■ Do I need medications for paranoia?

_____

_____

_____

_____

_____

Triggers

■ Turning to the wrong people and overwhelming them.
■ Argumentative people.
■ Medications that make me irritated.
■ Crowds.

_____

_____

_____

_____

_____

Asking for Help

- See a therapist for help with relationship problems.
- Ask friends and family to read this book so that they can understand me a bit better.
- Remember to ask for help from the right people.
- Join a support group.

_____

_____

_____

_____

_____

Lifestyle Changes I Can Make

- Use the chain of command for neediness.
- Teach others how to help me.
- Read books on relationships.
- Exercise more.

_____

_____

_____

_____

_____

Adele's Story

Age 40

I had a friend from high school that I really loved. She was fun and beautiful and I always wanted to be more like her. She got the guys and always took risks and did what she wanted. Then she changed. She got really clingy. Her depression got worse. She had always been depressed off and on, but this was ridiculous. She would stop by and just sit around. I didn't have time for this. I didn't want her to just drop by unannounced. It's not how I am. She would get upset if I went out with other people and when I told her I was busy, she would send me an e-mail and tell me I didn't really care about her. When I started to have some trouble with my relationship with my partner, she was so selfish! She didn't understand that *I* needed time to deal with my own life. One day she came over and I just couldn't help it. I told her not to come over anymore. She rushed out of the house and went home and took some pills. It's like your worst fear in the world that you will cause someone to do this. But I realize that I didn't cause anything. I loved her the best I could. She survived and is a lot better. A lot better. But things were never the same between us. She was so needy I couldn't do what she wanted anymore.

LOSS OF HOPE

Hopelessness is a totally normal bipolar disorder feeling. It's part of the illness and is one of the main symptoms of depression. When you feel hopeless, it really doesn't help if people in

■ *For Family and Friends*

Be careful not to forget what you have learned in previous chapters. When your loved one is hopeless, pointing out all that he or she has to live for, including your love, will not work. Dealing with the bipolar disorder that causes the loss of hope is the only way to get through to someone who is depressed because of a downswing.

your life point out all the good things you have going. Bipolar disorder won't let you listen to what they say. Instead, it helps if you can see hopelessness as a sign that you need help managing the illness. Use the following section to create a plan for ending the hopeless feelings.

Symptoms

- Saying things like, "I don't see any reason to keep living like this."
- Starting all-or-nothing thinking: "Nothing will ever be better. I'll always be this way. Life will always be terrible."
- Asking, "What's the point?"
- Feeling that this illness has ruined my life forever.

_____

_____

_____

_____

_____

Medications

- Medications don't seem to be working.
- I don't have the money for all the medications I need.
- I don't see the point in taking medications.
- I don't take medications.

_____

_____

_____

_____

_____

Triggers

- Isolating myself and drinking alcohol alone.
- Relationship problems.

- Poor diet and no exercise.
- Medication problems.

_____

_____

_____

_____

_____

Asking for Help

- Find a support group.
- Teach others how to respond to me when I say hopeless things.
- Look into government assistance for medications.
- Find a doctor who can help me get my medications regulated.

_____

_____

_____

_____

Lifestyle Changes I Can Make

- Start doing the things I love again—even if I don't feel like it.
- Join a group of like-minded people.
- Recognize my leading comments and see them as a sign that I'm sick.
- Try the tips in this book.

_____

_____

_____

_____

■ *For Family and Friends*

How do you feel when your loved one loses all hope? It can be incredibly scary, but the more you can remember that loss of hope is a typical bipolar disorder symptom, the easier it will be for you to get your loved one the help that's so crucial. Loss of hope may not make any sense if you see that the person's life is filled with love and interesting things to do. But none of this matters to bipolar disorder. Love has never been a cure for bipolar disorder mood swings, just as love is never a cure for diabetes. Loss of hope is a symptom of this illness and needs to be treated aggressively.

Karl's Story

Age 50

I often wake up in the morning with the thought, *What's the point?* This is a terrible way to wake up. It's like I don't even get a chance to have a good day. The feeling doesn't stop there. I then think, *Is this all there is to life? We get up. Eat breakfast. Go to work. Talk with people. Eat lunch. Talk with people. Eat dinner. Go to bed.* It just all seems so unbelievably depressing. There *must* be more to life. What is it? Do happy people do more things? I think their lives are a lot better than mine. They laugh and go places and get stimulation and excitement and have better relationships. My life just feels so pointless and I know that it will always be like this. I have no hope for my future at all.

The above is the old me talking. Things are different now for one reason: I don't listen to the talk anymore. I still hear it and often wake up with the *What is the point?* thought. It's still there. I still feel incredibly hopeless. But I now know it can't possibly be real because I feel it no matter where I am in life and I only hear it when I'm depressed. When I'm not depressed I just wake up and get on with my day and often enjoy myself! I hate bipolar disorder because it does this to me, but I manage it now. I talk back and say, *My life is what it is and I make it what it is and that is my purpose and that is the point.* This helps a lot and I'm much, much happier.

GETTING THINGS DONE WHEN YOU'RE DEPRESSED

It often feels impossible to get things done when you're depressed. For many people, it's a struggle to get out of bed, much less do the work that needs to be done in a day. This is normal. Most people with depression have trouble getting things done. It's a symptom of the illness, and you're not alone if you feel unmotivated when you're depressed. One of the best ways to deal with this problem is to have a plan ready and waiting that you can use as soon as the depression starts. Use the following section to create a plan you can use on the days you need an extra push to get things done.

Symptoms

- Saying things like, "I just don't have the energy to do anything."
- Feeling overwhelmed with all I have to do, so I do nothing.
- Feeling that the steps of a project are insurmountable.
- Feeling that my brain is totally scattered.

_____

_____

_____

_____

_____

■ *For Family and Friends*

There is little more frustrating for family members and friends than to watch someone sit around and never get anything done. And yet the reality of depression is that it often makes it impossible for your loved one to get anything done. It's as though the brain stops working. For some people, even putting one foot in front of the other is too much work. The only way to help your loved one treat this inertia is to offer a reminder that it's a symptom of depression, and to make sure he or she has a plan in place for the moment symptoms start.

Medications

- My medications make me really tired all the time.
- My medications dull my brain and I often feel blank.
- I can try a new medication that can help with my energy level.
- I can talk with my doctor about my medications.

_____

_____

_____

_____

_____

Triggers

- Staying in bed all day.
- Poor diet and no exercise.
- Taking on too much.
- Feeling that work is too stressful.

_____

_____

_____

_____

_____

Asking for Help

- Ask the people in my life to help me around the house.
- Ask someone to help me get organized.
- Get tips from a therapist.
- Ask someone to sit with me and encourage me as I do a task.

_____

_____

_____

_____

_____

Lifestyle Changes I Can Make

- Praise myself when I take the first step of a project.
- Create really small to-do lists and then get them done.
- Exercise to create energy.
- Decide to do things even when I don't feel like doing them.

_____

_____

_____

_____

_____

Julie's Story

Age 42

Before I was diagnosed with bipolar disorder, I actually went through years where I couldn't seem to get anything done. The ideas were in my head, but execution of these ideas was not possible. Actually, the ideas *were* executed! They died before they went anywhere. I used to make these huge lists of all I had to do. I remember one list:

Wake up and do yoga
Make a healthy breakfast
Finish grant proposal
Study some French
Take a walk
Clean apartment

What makes this really ridiculous is that I couldn't do any of it. It's like my brain could make the list, but it couldn't get moving. Anyway, that list was too much for a normal person. I got down on myself for years for not being productive. Then I realized that depression makes it impossible to get things done. That it's normal for all people with depression and if you want to get something done, you don't wait until you want to do it. You have to just do it even when it feels impossible. This breaks the cycle. It worked for me. I set one goal per day and then got it done. Sometimes it was getting out of bed! Then it got better. I got more work done. I was easier on myself. Depression will never want to get anything done, but I do. So I do it. I was often depressed when I wrote this book. But I had my plan and I used it and I finished the book.

BRAIN RACING AND LOOPING

Brain racing and looping happen when your brain seems to go into high gear and just won't turn off. You can hear the same song over and over again or constantly replay a conversation in your head. You can hear numbers, such as *1, 2, 3, 4, 5—1, 2, 3, 4, 5* . . . Brain racing and looping are often a sign that you're overstimulated or psychotic. They're also a sign that you need to stop what you're doing and examine your lifestyle. Use the following section to help you figure out what causes your brain racing and looping and what you can do in the future to prevent it. Some studies show that writing down these thoughts may help stop the looping. Keep this in mind as you fill out this exercise.

Symptoms

■ Saying things like, "My brain just won't turn off."
■ Hearing music in my brain that won't stop playing.
■ Continually hearing an old conversation in my head, over and over again—especially an imagined or worrisome conversation.
■ Feeling like my brain keeps running even when I'm sleeping.

_____

_____

_____

_____

_____

Medications

■ My new medication is causing problems.
■ My antidepressant is overstimulating.
■ My medications need adjusting and I want to talk to my doctor about my constant brain activity. Do I need an antipsychotic until this calms down?
■ I stopped my medications.

_____

_____

_____

_____

_____

Triggers

- ▪ Caffeine, other stimulants.
- ▪ Lack of sleep.
- ▪ Arguments.
- ▪ Wondering, *Am I manic?*

_____

_____

_____

_____

Asking for Help

- ▪ Ask the people in my life to help limit stimulation in my environment.
- ▪ Ask my doctor about my medications.
- ▪ Ask if anyone has techniques to quiet the brain.
- ▪ Ask my support group for their advice.

_____

_____

_____

_____

▪ *For Family and Friends*

Brain racing and looping is a very uncomfortable part of bipolar disorder. It affects sleep and often leaves your loved one unable to concentrate. It's as though the brain takes over like a skipping record and just keeps saying the same thing again and again.

Lifestyle Changes I Can Make

- Stop caffeine.
- Go to sleep at a regular time.
- Exercise more, especially relaxing exercises such as yoga that involve calming breathing.
- Turn off the television.

_____

_____

_____

_____

_____

Bob's Story

Age 29

One night when I was lying in bed, I tried to count all the thoughts going on in my head. I heard sections of songs that would repeat over and over again. I heard pieces of conversations I had earlier that day. I felt worries moving around. I was making a to-do list. I then started to think about thinking about all that was going on in my head. It sounded like a lot of feedback. John Lennon wrote a song called "Revolution #9." That song is the closest thing I've ever heard that describes what it's like to have a brain that won't turn off. It can be really terrible. It's hard to sleep. You can't choose your own thoughts. It takes time to make it stop. It's scary sometimes. I knew I had to make a lot of changes. I stopped caffeine. I started by changing to decaf and then stopped it all. It was hard, but it calmed my mind down at least a little bit. I limited my activities before bed. I talked to my doctor about sleep medications and antianxiety medications. I really tried to make more choices that reflected what I wanted to do instead of just blindly doing what bipolar disorder wanted me to do. Sometimes this new life feels very boring. I also have trouble not falling back into old behavior. But I definitely feel better, and on more and more nights I have a lot less thoughts and definitely sleep better. It's a tradeoff, but it's worth it.

SEXUAL PROBLEMS

Sexual problems are common with bipolar disorder. From a lack of sexuality when you're depressed to hypersexuality when you're manic, bipolar disorder can make your sex life really miserable. Then there are the medication side effects to complicate the problem. It's important that you separate how you behaved sexually before medications, as well as how you feel sexually when you're well, from the way you feel sexually when you're sick and on meds. If you have a normal sex drive when you're well or if you enjoyed sex before you went on medications, then you can assume that the problems are bipolar-disorder-related. If you have always had sexual issues and bipolar disorder simply makes them worse, then you will approach the problem differently. Once again, treating bipolar disorder first so that you can find some stability is the best way to deal with sexual problems caused by the illness. Use the following section to help you create a plan for working on the sexual problems you may have.

Symptoms

- Saying things like, "I think I'm frigid/asexual."
- Wanting to have sex with multiple partners.
- Being unable to have an orgasm.
- Feeling no sexual desire.

_____

_____

_____

_____

Medications

- My antidepressant leaves me unable to have an orgasm.
- My medications make me feel dull, fat, and unsexy.
- My medications are overstimulating and I want more sex than normal.
- I stopped my medications.

_____

_____

_____

_____

_____

Triggers

- Weight gain.
- Medications.
- Mania/depression/psychosis.
- Relationship problems.

_____

_____

_____

_____

_____

Asking for Help

- Talk with a sex therapist who has experience with mental illness.
- Tell my doctor about my concerns and discuss medications.
- Ask my doctor for help in clarifying what is the bipolar disorder and what is me.
- Talk honestly with my partner.

_____

_____

_____

_____

_____

Lifestyle Changes I Can Make

- Exercise to increase endorphins and sexual desire.
- Get testosterone level checked (both men and women can do this).
- Decide what is the bipolar disorder and what is actually a relationship issue, and work on the relationship issues.
- Get help for weight loss.

_____

_____

_____

_____

_____

■ *For Family and Friends*

It is so easy to judge your loved one for inappropriate sexual behavior. It may be very hard for you to realize that this is a part of bipolar disorder for many people. Mania is especially notorious for ending all inhibitions—to the point that your loved one may do something that wrecks a relationship or transmits a serious disease. This is tragic in many ways, but unfortunately quite normal. The best defense against inappropriate sexual behavior is preventing the mood swings that cause the behavior.

Chris's Story

Age 40

How can I describe my sexual "issues" when it comes to bipolar disorder? Well, there's the manic sex that is often unprotected and very spur of the moment. I used to just go with my feelings on that one. Then there's the drunk sex where I hope the sex will make me feel more alive when I'm feeling dead inside. There is the impotent sex when I can't even get the energy to live, so I certainly don't have the energy for sex. Then there's the no-orgasm sex that comes with quite a few medications. Bipolar disorder has not been very kind to me sexually. It helped to finally realize that if I deal with the bipolar disorder, there is really a chance that my sex life will get more normal and enjoyable. I changed a few things at first. I talked honestly with my partner about what the illness was doing to me and how we could work together to manage the mood swings so I would have the energy to be sexual. I talked with my doctor about my meds. I walked a lot more. It helped my moods. I also wrote down my thoughts before I got manic and made poor sexual decisions. Things are a lot better. As I focused more on treating the illness and less on my sexual "problems," things got calmer and I felt more sexual immediately.

IRRITATION, ANGER, AND AGGRESSION

Irritation, anger, and aggression are often seen as personality problems instead of bipolar disorder problems, but they're actually very common bipolar disorder symptoms. Whether caused by depression or mania, irritation, anger, and aggression can create serious difficulties in your life if they're not treated effectively. These feelings are often a sign that you need to examine your lifestyle and figure out what is triggering the behaviors. Use the following section to create a plan for stopping these destructive symptoms from ruining your life.

Symptoms

- Saying things like, "People are so stupid!"
- Feeling like hitting or kicking something or someone.
- Getting so angry that I feel I'm going to explode!
- Having road rage/extreme impatience.
- Stabbing someone, or thinking of stabbing someone.

_____

_____

_____

_____

_____

Medications

- My new medication is making me irritable.
- I stopped my medications because they were making me feel slow.
- My medications are not working.
- My medications make me feel antsy.

_____

_____

_____

_____

_____

Triggers

- Alcohol/drugs/caffeine.
- Going to a busy event at work, attending a social event, or visiting a crowded restaurant. Hanging out at a bar.
- People (especially my kids) wanting too much from me.
- Vacation.

■ *For Family and Friends*

Family members and friends are often on the receiving end of an irritation and anger mood swing. Sometimes they are the ones who get hit. This is where bipolar disorder behavior in your loved one can actually endanger your life. The milder version of the anger can be treated successfully, but the rage and violence that sometimes come with a mood swing—especially if drugs or alcohol are involved—may be too tough for you to treat without outside help.

_____

_____

_____

_____

_____

Lewis's Story

Age 27

Before I got it under control, my anger used to make me feel good. Or I should say that acting on my anger made me feel good. Imagine a pot filled with water. As it starts to boil, the lid has to come up a bit to let the steam out. When I'm angry because of bipolar disorder, there is no loss of steam. That lid just sits there and I boil and boil and boil and then I do something to get all that anger out of me and I actually feel a lot, lot better. That lid is gone! The steam is out! I've punched a cop. I've broken my hand on a wall. I've tried to choke a friend. I've been in jail. What else . . . I've had road rage so bad I made a guy pull over so I could fight him. Luckily he drove off.

Asking for Help

- ▪ Teach people to respond to my symptoms instead of reacting to them.
- ▪ Talk with my doctor about a medication change.
- ▪ Ask friends and family to be patient with me.
- ▪ Join a support group.

_____

_____

_____

_____

_____

Lifestyle Changes I Can Make

- ▪ Make a deal with myself not to take out my irritation or anger on others.
- ▪ Take a walk the minute I start to feel irritated.
- ▪ Work on my diet/stop caffeine. Get real about alcohol.
- ▪ Really learn to notice the very first signs of irritation so that it doesn't turn into something more serious.

_____

_____

_____

_____

_____

NEGATIVE SELF-TALK

Negative self-talk is a common symptom of depression. It's as though your brain is offering a running commentary on everything you do wrong and how you'll never succeed. As you read in the introduction, sometimes the talk you hear is actually an hallucination or an intrusive thought and is caused by psychosis. For many people, negative self-talk happens after a stressful event, though it can be chronic as well. This negative self-talk can be very destructive—it may cause you not to reach your goals and can affect your relationships adversely. Use the following section to create a plan for managing and ultimately preventing negative self-talk.

Symptoms

- Saying things like, "I hate myself."
- Feeling negative about myself and being unable to think anything positive about myself.
- Putting myself down in front of others because it's what I hear in my head.
- Feeling negative about other people as well.

_____

_____

_____

_____

_____

Medications

- I can talk to my doctor about these negative thoughts.
- Antidepressants can help with the depression and help stop the negative thinking.
- I stopped my medications because I don't have any money.
- The medications make me unhappier than before.

_____

_____

_____

_____

_____

Triggers

- Stressful events, including trauma and arguments.
- Stress at work or school.
- Nonaccepting people in my life.
- Situations I can't control, which often make me talk negatively about myself and others.

_____

_____

_____

_____

_____

Asking for Help

- Find a therapist who can help me with cognitive therapy techniques.
- Ask others to point out when I talk negatively about myself so that I can say something positive about myself.
- Ask my doctor for ideas.
- Reach out to the happy, stable people in my life.

_____

_____

_____

_____

_____

Lifestyle Changes You Can Make

- Work on diet and exercise to improve the depression and improve my thoughts.
- Avoid the stressful people and events that I know make me sick.
- Praise myself no matter what I do and make a rule that I can't put myself down anymore.
- Say no to the thoughts and remind myself that it's the depression talking.

■ *For Family and Friends*

As you learned in the bipolar conversation chapter, trying to talk someone out of negative thinking is pointless. What works is addressing the role depression plays in negative thinking and then learning to respond to what your loved one says with something constructive. You can also create a negative-free zone. When your loved one is negative, say, "I like to focus on your positive qualities." This may make your loved one angry at first, but keep trying. It may help him or her see that the negative talk is attributable to bipolar disorder and not some personal failing.

Karen's Story

Age 32

This is what I used to hear when I tried to sing. "You can't sing. What makes you think you can sing? Who are *you* kidding? Do you think you're some big kind of star? You're off key and you'll make a fool of yourself. When you sing you go flat. People are looking at you funny when you sing. Singing is for professionals. Look how they sound. You will never be that good. You're too old to learn to sing. No one is clapping. You sound crappy. You are boring people. Karaoke is not singing! You took voice lessons when you were younger and you're still no good. Don't try to sing. Forget singing. Give it up. No way will it work. What songs anyway? Who will listen to you? Remember what your mother said? Everyone will be embarrassed. Stop! Don't even think of singing." Can you question why I never sang until I was diagnosed and learned to treat and ignore the voices?

CULTURAL ISSUES

You may come from a background where mental illness is seen as something personal. Maybe your family doesn't discuss mental illness. Maybe your culture believes it's a sign of weakness. Whatever the case, your cultural background can cause extra stress when it comes to treating bipolar disorder, especially if your family doesn't speak the same language as your doctors and therapists. They may feel confused, or wonder what you have done wrong to cause all these troubles to the family. This can cause considerable pressure on you at a time when you need to focus on your own health. Use the following section to help you create a plan for living within your culture while still getting the help you need to treat bipolar disorder.

Symptoms

- I feel pressured to be what my culture wants me to be.
- In my culture, women are supposed to be strong.
- My parents don't believe in bipolar disorder.
- Mental illness is taboo in my culture and is seen as a spirit problem.
- Men are not mentally ill in my culture.

_____

_____

_____

_____

_____

Medications

- Medications are something weak people take.
- I have to learn to accept that I need medications and not let my family influence my decisions.
- I have to hide my medications.
- My family doesn't understand my weight gain.

_____

_____

_____

_____

_____

Triggers

- My friends and family members make me feel weak for being sick.
- My friends and family tell me it's all in my head, and this is terribly stressful.
- I can't turn to my family for help.
- The stress over this issue makes me more ill.

_____

_____

_____

_____

Asking for Help

- See a therapist from my own culture who understands what I'm going through.
- Look within Internet chat groups for people in similar situations.
- Ask my doctor for help.
- Turn to people who do not judge me.
- Get someone who can speak my parents' language to explain bipolar disorder medically.

_____

_____

_____

_____

_____

■ *For Family and Friends*

Were you raised in a culture where mental illness was seen as a weakness? Is there a chance that you have passed this attitude on to your loved one? This illness is serious enough without worrying about the cultural pressure that many family members—often older ones—put on the person with bipolar disorder. If you see a family member or friend telling your loved one that she's not really sick and that she needs to just get her act together, maybe you can gently remind him that bipolar disorder—like diabetes—is an illness, not a personal failing.

Lifestyle Changes I Can Make

- Discuss my illness with people who understand.
- Talk with my family about other issues, and save bipolar disorder for my health care professionals.
- Ask my friends and family to read this book, ask for their questions, and explain that bipolar disorder is a physical illness.
- Accept my culture, but also educate my friends and family members.

_____

_____

_____

_____

Angela's Story

Age 46

I'm a black woman and in my family black women are stronnnnnggggg. We don't break down. We hold the family together. We're the matriarchs. We don't cry or let others get us down. When I got diagnosed I felt so weak. I used to cry all the time. I thought, *What role will I play in the family now?* I identified so much with my family strength and how I got everyone through things. How would people think of me now? Would they tell me to just snap out of it? Would they say, *Strong women don't get mental illnesses?* I thought about this so much it made me even sicker. Things got better when I accepted that I have an illness, not a weakness. I learned what to say to every single person who seemed to judge me for needing so much help. I said, "If I had cancer, would you say this to me? If I had some other serious illness, like pneumonia, would you tell me to get more energy and clean my house better?" This stops people really quickly and makes them think. I told many of the people who did understand that they would have to say this for me when they heard others talk or truly not understand this illness. Once I made it clear that I have an illness, I started to teach them about my own mood swings. Not everyone changed. I know my father struggles with all the feelings he had before I was finally diagnosed. But I have faith he will change as well.

SUICIDAL THOUGHTS

As scary as they are, suicidal thoughts are a normal part of bipolar disorder. They mean that you're sick and need help. They don't mean that life is worthless or that you need to die. They mean that bipolar disorder is in control and that you're not thinking rationally. Do you have active thoughts in which you actually plan what you will do? Or do you have more passive thoughts where you just think about dying? When do you have these suicidal thoughts? Do they happen after an argument? Are they stress-related? The more aware you are of what causes the suicidal thoughts, the easier it will be to prevent them.

If you have suicidal thoughts, talk about them openly. Explain to family members and friends that they're a normal part of bipolar disorder and are a sign that you need help and

◼ *For Family and Friends*

This is naturally the most dangerous part of bipolar disorder. It's scary for a family member or friend to see suicidal behavior, and it's really scary when you hear your loved one say he or she wants to die. As noted, as scary as this is, suicidal thoughts are a normal part of bipolar disorder and must be treated aggressively with medications and help from a trained health care professional. If you feel your loved one is going to take action, you will need to get him or her to the hospital immediately, despite any protests. Yes, this is hard. It's sometimes so difficult you may feel you won't live through it yourself, but you can. You need tools ready and in place for if and when suicidal thoughts do happen, and you need to be prepared to ask "Are you suicidal?" as soon as you see the warning signs. So many family members and friends are shocked at suicide—it's often very easy for the suicidal person to hide his or her feelings. But there are early warning signs, such as giving away possessions, crying all day, becoming aggressive, and engaging in very, very risky behaviors as well as saying, "You would be better off without me." It's also important to know that someone who is suicidal can appear calm and silent before actually taking action. Don't wait until it's too late to help your loved one.

support. If you're having suicidal thoughts regularly, it's very important that you talk with your doctor immediately. It means that you're sick and need help. *People with bipolar disorder resort to suicidal behavior to relieve the pain of mood swings; it doesn't mean they want to end their lives.* Antipsychotics, as well as other bipolar disorder medications, can often work miracles with suicidal thoughts. Instead of trying to kill yourself, say to yourself, *This is an illness and I'm going to see a doctor first for help.* You won't want to do this, but you must. Suicide ends the pain, but it also ends your life—and that's not a good tradeoff. There are other and better ways to end the pain caused by bipolar disorder. When you deal with the pain caused by the mood swings, you will have a lot more desire to live.

Symptoms

- Saying things like, "I wish I were dead."
- "Things would be easier if I wrecked my car and died."
- "I could get a hose to put in my exhaust, shut the windows of my car, and just go to sleep."
- "I just don't think I can live with this pain anymore."
- Hearing a voice: "Jump off that bridge."

_____

_____

_____

_____

Medications

- My new medication started the thoughts (I need to see my doctor immediately).
- My medications aren't working.
- I must talk with my doctor about antipsychotic medications for suicidal thoughts.
- I need to ask about my options.

_____

_____

_____

_____

Triggers

- Breakup of a relationship.
- Trouble at work.
- Fights with people I love.
- Watching upsetting media.

_____

_____

_____

_____

_____

Asking for Help

■ Tell my doctor I'm having suicidal thoughts, even though I'm scared and embar-
rassed and really do believe things would be better if I were dead.
■ Tell my friends that I'm sick, and ask for their help.
■ Make sure I talk with the right people.
■ Find a person to call who can listen.

_____

_____

_____

_____

_____

Lifestyle Changes I Can Make

■ Avoid arguments and stressful people.
■ Exercise more/watch my diet.
■ Keep my life balanced.
■ Constantly remind myself that these thoughts do not mean I have to act on them.
They mean that I'm sick and need help for bipolar disorder.

_____

_____

_____

_____

_____

Sharine's Story

Age 28

I tried to kill myself when I was fourteen years old. I remember being so numb that all I wanted to do was get away and not have to feel this way anymore. I heard voices that said, "You'll be better off dead. Take the pills. You can just take all the pills at once. This is the best thing. Nothing will ever get better." Everything in the world felt hopeless: school, the guy I liked, my girlfriends. I didn't care about reading or movies like I used to. I stopped talking on the phone. I watched so much television. My parents were always on my case. I never told them what was happening. I now know that they thought I was just being a teenager. If I had it to do over again, I would tell my parents that the thoughts I was having had nothing to do with my age. I felt this strange compulsion to really kill myself. I thought about it for months and soon it was all I thought about. It was like something was pulling me by this really strong rope. It was impossible for me to fight. It seemed like the right thing to do. I was sure the world would be a better place without me. It would feel good to be gone and healthy again. I know that sounds crazy, but I just hurt so much in my brain. I'm truly thankful I lived. I got help. It was a pretty shocking wake-up call for my parents. I'm sorry to say that they were clueless, but they were. This has a lot to do with me. I simply didn't tell them what was going on. I wasn't lying. The thoughts were just too secretive and strong. I think there were a lot of signs they missed. I never tried to kill myself again. The meds really changed my life. I still get the thoughts, but I know they aren't real. I tell my parents and everyone about them now. My friends even understand bipolar disorder a lot better.

UNDERSTANDING THAT PLANS MAKE A DIFFERENCE

Many of the problems covered in this chapter arise when bipolar disorder is not being treated effectively. As you use the 4-Step Plan in this book, you may find that many of the problems you currently experience get better as a natural result of managing the illness successfully. That is the goal. The exercises in this chapter are a good first step to preventing the problems from happening over and over again, and they have given you a framework to use each time a new situation arises that you feel you can't control. Remember, if a chapter in a book can outline many of the problems you experience because of bipolar disorder, this shows you that it's an illness. Everyone with the illness has similar problems. And illnesses can be treated.

Your Toolbox

Knowledge about bipolar disorder.

A correct diagnosis.

A list of your major symptoms.

Medication knowledge.

Help with side effects.

A regular sleep schedule.

A bipolar-friendly diet.

A daily walk.

Regular and appropriate bright light exposure.

A clear picture of your work history.

A clear picture of your current financial position.

A list of your bipolar disorder triggers.

Tips to modify and stop the triggers.

The ability to recognize the bipolar conversation.

A list of leading comments and actions.

The ability to respond instead of reacting to your own bipolar disorder language.

A supportive health care team.

Well-planned appointments.

Friends and family members who can help.

Outside sources of support.

A plan to prevent hospital visits.

Specific plans for problems caused by bipolar disorder.

The Take Charge 4-Step Treatment Plan.

CHAPTER 11

PLANNING FOR THE FUTURE

Now that you have a better idea of how to use the Take Charge 4-Step Treatment Plan to help you manage bipolar disorder effectively, what is the next step? Where do you want to go with this information? As you know, bipolar disorder is a very difficult illness to manage. It can catch you unawares and lead you back into old behaviors very quickly. If you want to prevent this from happening in your future, it will help if you get started now with some of the ideas in this book. Filling out the charts in the appendix is a good way to begin, as is using the journal. The important thing to remember is that creating a future that is not controlled by bipolar disorder symptoms may take some time, but it is definitely possible.

This chapter covers some of the areas that may get in the way of your using the 4-Step Treatment Plan outlined in this book, as well as offering some tips on how to prevent the illness from affecting your future the way it has affected your past. Finally, the chapter encourages you to keep going and to give yourself time to make the changes you want and need to make in order to stay stable.

PREPARING FOR A BRIGHTER FUTURE

If bipolar disorder has created chaos in your past, you may welcome the thought that your future can be more stable. You can make choices now that ensure a future you'll look forward to. It really is about the choices you make when you are well. The more prevention you can do during the stable times, the more able you will be to recognize, treat, and end the mood swings before they go too far. The following section will offer tips on how you can create a future that focuses on you and what you want from life instead of a future spent in crisis because of bipolar disorder.

Accepting the Diagnosis

One of the main obstacles you may face in the future is accepting the diagnosis of bipolar disorder. It's not as though you have an illness that can be treated once, whereupon you go back to a regular life. So many people with bipolar disorder struggle with accepting the reality of a lifetime mental illness. Another complication is that once a mood swing goes too far, it can lead to poor judgment—by telling you that you don't need medications, for instance, or that the diagnosis isn't real and you don't really have the illness. Decisions are then made based on the poor judgment caused by bipolar disorder, and lives are ruined once again. One way to prevent this is to acknowledge right now, as you read this book, that you need to work on accepting the bipolar disorder diagnosis—and that it's normal if it takes years to become truly accepting. If you go back and forth on what you think— *Maybe the diagnosis is a mistake. Maybe it will go away. Maybe everyone is wrong*—then you're only fighting with your health and future. It serves no purpose. Acceptance has

■ *For Family and Friends*

Family members and friends can also have a hard time accepting that their loved one has a serious mental illness. You had dreams yourself. If your partner is diagnosed, your dreams of traveling together may change significantly. As a parent, your dreams for your child may have to change when it comes to school and work. Siblings may get less attention. Friends may not get to socialize with their friend as much. In fact, so many things can change for the person with bipolar disorder that it's easier to deny reality than accept that *you* may have to change as well. And yet, as with many big changes, people acclimate. Lives may have to change, but they often change for the better. Communication can become more effective, families can become closer, and the person with the illness can get better care and understanding now that he or she is diagnosed. There is hope.

nothing to do with giving in to bipolar disorder. What it means is that you're willing to say the following to yourself, then go on from there:

I have a serious mental illness that I will have to manage for the rest of my life. I need medications for this illness. There is a good chance that I'll get sick again, and if life is especially stressful I'll probably get sick quite often. There's also a very good chance that manic thoughts will tell me that I'm fine and the people around me are crazy. I may get suicidal. I need help from friends and family to manage this illness. I accept that I need a health care team to help me manage my medications and other treatment options. I may hate this illness and what it does to my life, but I want to accept reality so that I don't spend my energy fighting something I can't change. I want to save my energy for managing the illness effectively so that I can lead a happy and stable life.

Creating New Dreams and Goals

A bipolar disorder diagnosis may feel like a death sentence to your hopes and dreams, but it doesn't have to be that way. There is no question that many of your dreams and goals will have to be modified, and that some of them will have to be let go of, but once you use a comprehensive treatment plan that helps you manage the illness successfully, you can get back to your dreams and goals with pleasure. They may be different than you'd planned on, but they can be just as rewarding. This may seem impossible now, but just keep going. It gets better.

Knowing the Signs That You're Getting Sick

As said in many of the chapters, knowing the first signs that you're getting sick and teaching others to look for these signs as well is one of the most powerful ways to prevent bipolar disorder mood swings from taking over your life. This simple tool can help your future remain focused on health instead of on treating out-of-control mood swings.

Taking Care of Bipolar Disorder in the Present

Bipolar disorder has a way of sneaking up on you. If you can remind yourself to be present at all times and look for the signs that you're starting a mood swing, you can stop many of your serious episodes before they even get to the second stage. The journal at the

Alberto's Story

Age 46

It took me about seven years to really come to terms with bipolar disorder. I kept hoping it would just go away. Maybe it was like a really bad virus and all I needed to find was the drug that would get rid of the virus. I know I was superhard on myself for years because I couldn't seem to get my act together. It was such a loss to realize that this is my life, for the rest of my life. It's not going to go away. I can learn to manage it. I can be an optimist when it comes to treatment, but I'm not going to wake up one day and be "cured." For a long time I would wake up in the morning and think, *Maybe today's the day that I will wake up and I won't have bipolar disorder anymore.* Or I would wake up and think, *Oh, my God. I have bipolar disorder. Nothing will ever get better.* But it does get better. Year after year I manage my symptoms more successfully, and each year is better than the last. I really do stick to my treatment plan—usually. I still have tough days, but that's a lot better than having tough years and ending up in the hospital. I don't go to the hospital anymore and I am so proud of myself for that. My depressions are much shorter now and as long as I stay on my meds and watch my lifestyle I don't get too manic. I think that management means accepting where I am and then going easy on myself every day that I do my best. Life is good now. I'm a good father. I'm better. So much better than before I was diagnosed. I accept where I am today. I still get this twinge of hope that it's all a dream, but I find that the more I live in the reality of the fact that I have a mental illness, the more proud I am of my considerable accomplishment of staying alive and creating a really good life.

end of this book can help you manage the illness daily, so that you don't end up back in the hospital with no idea why. The more you monitor your moods and behaviors, the better chance you have of preventing a serious episode.

Recognizing Your Personal Bipolar Disorder Wake-Up Call

Each person has a different wake-up call, signaling that bipolar disorder is taking over his or her life. What is yours? Is it an increase in spending? Dependency on drugs, alcohol, or food? Sleep problems? Think of the signs that start each of your major bipolar disorder symptoms. Write your personal wake-up calls here so that you will know that you need to take action and treat bipolar disorder first instead of ignoring these signs and getting sick again.

Your Personal Wake-Up Calls

_____   _____

_____   _____

_____   _____

_____   _____

_____   _____

The Bipolar Disorder Check-In

The bipolar disorder check-in can be a lifesaver. It's a simple process that can help you manage the illness successfully so that an episode doesn't sneak up on you and ruin your life once again. The journal section of this book (appendix C) will help you with this process. The check-in works like this: Using a calendar, handheld organizer, friend, or even something like a weekly alarm on your watch, create a bipolar disorder check-in time where you stop what you're doing and ask yourself how you are on a scale of 1 to 10 in terms of mood swings. (A 1 means that you're stable; a 10, that you really need some help.) You will examine your thoughts, feelings, and behaviors to see if you're stable or in need of management. This is a great way to deal with relationship issues and money problems that come up because of the mood swings. You can ask yourself the following questions during your check-in:

- How is my sleep?
- Am I eating a bipolar-friendly diet?
- Am I irritated?
- Am I depressed?
- Am I showing signs of mania?
- How is my spending?
- Am I having voice hallucinations or intrusive thoughts?

- Are people acting concerned about me?
- How are my relationships?

Letting Go of the Past

Learning to live with a serious lifelong illness takes an adjustment. It means that you have to look at your life differently—maybe quite differently—than you expected. One way to do this is to carefully examine all that you have lost in the past because of this illness, grieve for it, and then say that you're ready and willing to manage the illness in the present so that the grief of the past can be healed. This diagnosis is a loss. A big loss. The brain you thought would be there when you need it often malfunctions and wrecks your life. The body you thought would take care of you gets sick easily. This is very sad, and you may feel hopeless about your chances of getting well. Have you let people know what a challenge and burden it is to live with this illness every day? How can you come to terms with the reality of this illness so that you can move forward in health and joy? Talking about the feelings you have surrounding your diagnosis with a trusted person is a positive first step in learning to live with bipolar disorder without it taking over your life.

HOW SICK ARE YOU?

Sometimes it's hard to tell if your emotions are your own or if they are manufactured by bipolar disorder. This can be a real problem if your feelings are telling you to do some-

■ *For Family and Friends*

You can create your own check-in list. How are you feeling about bipolar disorder? Are you doing too much caretaking? Are you frustrated with how slowly things are changing? Do you see signs that your loved one is getting sick? This may seem like too much work at first, but the more you learn your loved one's specific behaviors around each symptom, the easier it becomes. The future can and often is more positive than you can even imagine. People, even those who have had very serious hospital visits, can return to everyday life.

thing drastic such as leave a job or a relationship. The following list will help you to determine if you're well and making decisions that you truly want to make, or are ill and need help with bipolar disorder before you take any serious steps. Whenever you're thinking of making a big change that will affect your future, read over the following list and resolve to make a decision from the real you and not the bipolar disorder you:

- Have you said this before and felt like this when you were sick in the past?
- When you consider yourself well, do you think this way?
- Is your thinking black and white, all or nothing?
- Do you think the real you is talking, or is it bipolar disorder talking?
- Are you thinking of making a snap decision?
- Do you tell yourself that you should have done things differently and that what you did do was all wrong?
- Are you unhappy in a relationship or a situation that has been quite happy in the past?
- Do you want to leave that relationship or situation because you know that things would be so much better if you were just left alone? Or do you want to leave because you know they would be much better off without you?
- Are your bipolar symptoms obvious to others but not to yourself?
- Are you lonely?
- Are you suddenly thinking of leaving a relationship because other people look like they are sexier and have more fun?
- Do you have thoughts such as: *Things would be better if I could just _____* or, *Things would be different if I could just _____*?
- Do you feel like quitting and canceling the things you love?
- Do your moods fluctuate? Do you feel that everything is terrible one minute, while the next minute you know things will be fine?
- Do things just feel all wrong?
- Does everything feel perfectly right, and you just know that this is the best decision in the world and it will change your life?

If you said yes to even a few of the items on the above list, there is a good chance you're sick. If a person has a bad cough, a high fever, and a terrible rash and decides to ignore all these symptoms in the hope that they will just go away, you would probably think he or she isn't being very smart. And yet people with bipolar disorder ignore their symptoms all the time and then wonder why they are so sick again. If any of the items on the above list ring true for you, this is the time to treat bipolar disorder first. It's not the time to make decisions based on faulty thinking. All good decisions can wait. Tell yourself that you will wait a week or two; if the feelings are just as strong, you will then take action on them. This will usually be very difficult as bipolar disorder behavior is so impulsive, but you can learn more control. In the meantime, focus on getting well so that you can make decisions that reflect the real you. Many people with bipolar disorder make decisions when they're sick that then affect their future in a very negative way. If you can remind yourself to use this checklist before you make a major decision, you may be able to prevent many of the situations that caused you trouble in the past.

The Take Charge 4-Step Treatment Plan is truly a circular, comprehensive way of treating bipolar disorder. You start with medications, change your lifestyle, learn to deal with the thoughts and behaviors caused by bipolar disorder, and then learn how to ask for help with the entire process. When you get ill, you can use the techniques from the plan over and over again to find stability. As you continue to follow this process, you will hopefully need fewer medications, be able to add some of the lifestyle choices you were not able to tolerate in the past, have fewer thought and behavior problems, and then need less help from the people around you. It is certainly a comprehensive and positive way to treat such a complicated illness.

Managing a serious illness takes practice. You will make mistakes. Sometimes they will be "real" mistakes (based on healthy decisions) and sometimes they will be bipolar-disorder-influenced mistakes. Stability may seem elusive if you are newly diagnosed and the mood swings are strong. But there is hope. By now you have most of the tools you need to manage this illness successfully, so that you can create a future that lets you enjoy

■ *For Family and Friends*

Never give up! Bipolar disorder is an illness that can be very effectively treated with the tools in this book. There *is* hope, and things *can* get better. With time and commitment, you can have a normal relationship with your loved one.

stable relationships, find useful and rewarding work, reach your dreams, and live the life you have always wanted. You really do have the tools you need to manage bipolar disorder. Whenever you need to refresh your management skills, you can come back to this book and remind yourself that you *can* manage this illness; all it takes is a plan.

Your Toolbox

You now have a toolbox full of ideas to help you manage bipolar disorder. You'll also find a journal and mood swing chart in appendix C to add to your collection. On the days when you feel overwhelmed and unable to cope with the challenges of this illness, get out this book and read the toolbox list in each chapter. This will remind you that you do have options in treating this illness. There *is* hope. You *can* get better and lead a happy, stable, and productive life.

You have the ability to take charge of bipolar disorder. You can't do it with medications only, and you can't do it alone. Never forget that you are the one who lives with the illness. Keep yourself well enough to have a clear enough brain to make your own decisions. Have a system in place to take care of you when your brain isn't well enough to take care of you.

RESOURCES

The following Web pages can help you find information on bipolar disorder, local support groups, and help with any questions you have regarding disability and your legal rights in your area.

Julie Fast's Bipolar Disorder Web Site
www.bipolarhappens.com

This site offers Julie's personal treatment plan, tips for managing the illness, a daily Web log, and a monthly newsletter that includes information for people with bipolar disorder as well as for their family members, friends, and health care professionals.

Julie Fast's Author Web Site
www.juliefast.com

This site offers up-to-date information on Julie's current work and public appearances.

National Alliance for the Mentally Ill
www.nami.org

This site offers help on where to find local branches of NAMI, and provides information on NAMI's services for consumers (people with bipolar disorder) as well as for friends and family members. NAMI's one thousand affiliates are dedicated to public education advocacy and support.

Depression and Bipolar Support Alliance
www.dbsalliance.org

This site offers information on bipolar disorder, support groups, and help for people with bipolar disorder as well as for friends and family members. The Web site includes screening tools, downloadable information brochures, a patient-to-patient doctor recommendation service, support group listings, open discussion boards, and live chat features. DBSA has more than a thousand peer-run support groups across the country.

Depression and Related Affective Disorders Association
www.drada.org

This site offers information on bipolar disorder and on support groups for consumers and their friends and family members.

Children and Adolescent Bipolar Foundation
www.cabf.org

This site is dedicated to support and education for families raising children with bipolar disorder.

SUGGESTED READING

Burns, David D. *Feeling Good: The New Mood Therapy.* New York: Avon, revised edition, 1999.

DesMaisons, Kathleen. *Potatoes Not Prozac.* New York: Simon & Schuster, 1999.

Fast, Julie A., and John D. Preston. *Loving Someone with Bipolar Disorder: Understanding and Helping Your Partner.* Oakland, CA: New Harbinger, 2004.

Preston, John D. *Lift Your Mood Now: Simple Things You Can Do to Beat the Blues.* Oakland, CA: New Harbinger, 2001.

Savona, Natalie. *The Kitchen Shrink: Foods and Recipes for a Healthy Mind.* London: Thorsons, 2003.

CHARTS AND JOURNAL PAGES

VISITS TO YOUR HEALTH CARE PROVIDER

Date/Time	Provider	What I Need to Bring	Questions to Ask

Make copies of this chart and fill in all the pertinent information on a separate sheet for each health care provider on your team.

HEALTH CARE PROVIDER CONTACT INFORMATION

Name: _____

Type of practice: _____

Name of practice/group: _____

Address: _____

Office phone: _____

Office fax: _____

Other office address: _____

Other office phone: _____

Office hours: _____

E-mail: _____

Web site: _____

Mobile/cell phone: _____

Contact person: _____

Office personnel: _____

Doctor(s): _____

Nurse(s): _____

Notes: _____

_____

_____

_____

_____

_____

_____

TRACK YOUR MEDICATIONS

Name of Drug	Date/Dose	Side Effects/Questions
_____	_____	_____
		_____
		_____
_____	_____	_____
		_____
		_____
_____	_____	_____
		_____
		_____
_____	_____	_____
		_____
		_____
_____	_____	_____
		_____
		_____
_____	_____	_____
		_____
		_____
_____	_____	_____
		_____
		_____

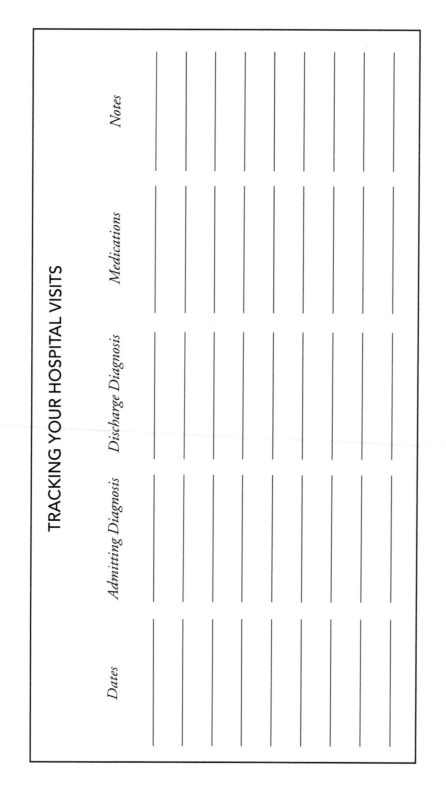

TRACKING YOUR HOSPITAL VISITS

Dates	Admitting Diagnosis	Discharge Diagnosis	Medications	Notes

PRIMARY INSURANCE CARRIER

Company name: _____

Member name: _____

Subscriber name: _____

Identification #: _____

Group #: _____

Kind of plan: _____

Plan/policy #: _____

Customer service phone: _____

Other phone numbers:

   Travel: _____

   Mental health: _____

   Percent/surgical services: _____

   Provider inquiry: _____

   Dental: _____

   Pharmacy provider: _____

Beginning and ending dates of coverage (MM/DD/YY): _____

Prescription plan: _____

Agent: _____

Phone: _____

Fax: _____

E-mail: _____

Web site: _____

(*Note:* You might be able to track your claim on the insurance company's Web site.)

Mail claims to: _____

Address: _____

City: _____

State: _____

Zip: _____

PRIMARY INSURANCE CO-PAYS

	In Network	*Out of Network*
Office visit	_____	_____
Emergency room	_____	_____
Urgent care	_____	_____
Rx formulary	_____	_____
Rx nonformulary	_____	_____
Inpatient	_____	_____
Outpatient	_____	_____
Mental health	_____	_____
Vision	_____	_____
Periodontist	_____	_____
Nutritionist	_____	_____
Exercise trainer	_____	_____
Neurologist	_____	_____
Emergency transport	_____	_____
Other	_____	_____

YOUR BIPOLAR DISORDER JOURNAL

You can begin using this journal system at any time. Once you've made copies of the pages provided and found a good system for keeping them together, fill in the dates, beginning with the date you start using the journal. These journal pages will help you to track your moods, and provide a space for you to use the ideas offered in this book.

The first goal when you start the journal is to look over the week and then list any bipolar-disorder-related appointments you may have. If there is a particular topic you want to cover in the appointment, write it under the time, and take your copied pages with you as a reminder to ask the questions you want answered. You can also make a list of any paperwork you need to get ready. There is a to-do list at the beginning of each week, where you can write any bipolar-disorder-related tasks you need to accomplish for the week, such as making an appointment, refilling a prescription, or asking for help. You will also notice that each day of the week asks you to look at a particular element in managing bipolar disorder.

At the end of each week is a place for you to think ahead regarding any possible triggers in the week you may need to prepare for. Think about travel, a work/school obligation, a social event, or any other change that may cause mood swings if you aren't prepared.

You may also want a separate journal that you use for writing your feelings and experiences in more detail. A journal can be a friend and confidant when the illness needs more help than the people around you can provide.

Sample Journal Pages

To do: Week of *01/01* to *01/07*
Call social worker, get antidepressant refilled. New antipsychotic? Look into gym? Review Take Charge *chapters. Call about the hospital bills.*

Monday, *01/01* (On a scale of 1–10, how is my mood?)
I'm not feeling too well today. I need more help than I'm getting. I'm going to try the tips in this book. I have to get better. I can't live like this anymore. My mood is a 3. I want to feel normal again. It's hard to get things done.

Tuesday, *01/02* (Are my medications working?)
Therapist 1 PM. I will talk with her about these medications. It just seems like I have to take so many drugs. How can I accept this? I just want to stop everything. I now know this is a sign that I need help. I will talk with Dr. J about the meds on Friday.

Wednesday, _01/03_ (How is my spending going this week?)
I'm worried about money. I can tell that I'm spending to feel better when I'm down. I'm worried about rent and need to talk to my social worker about getting some assistance. I missed so much work when I was in the hospital. It feels like I'll never recover.

Thursday, _01/04_ (Am I eating a bipolar-friendly diet?)
I'm trying! It's so hard when I feel so tired. I crave junk to get some energy. I am going to use the ideas in chapter 2 to make some changes. I have to remember that just one change is enough for now.

Friday, _01/05_ (How is my exercise this week?)
Dr. J, 3 PM. Ask about meds, weight gain, and if she knows a self-help group I can go to. We may try a new antidepressant.
I actually walked in the sun this morning and it really helped. I'm going to ask people to walk with me. I walk farther and it really helps my mood if I'm with a friend. I tried to remind myself about the serotonin and why I need to walk and move my arms and get sun in my eyes.

Saturday, _01/06_ (What can I do for fun today?)
I had a great morning. I'm finally feeling better. I pray it isn't mania. How do I know? I need to list my mania symptoms so that I can tell the difference between the real me and mania. I'm having tea with a friend for fun today. I'll try not to talk too much.

Sunday, _01/07_ (How was my sleep this week?)
I'm sleeping less. I know this is a sign. I can't get manic again. I just can't. I will try to sleep more tonight. Do I need to call Dr. J? I will see how much I sleep tonight. Could the new medication do this already?

Possible triggers this week: *There's a new person at work. This is stressful for me. The days are dark in the afternoon. I'm running out of money. My mother comes to visit in a few weeks and we always argue. What can I do now to make sure I don't get sick this time?*

You can make copies of the following pages to make sure you have enough for a few months.

JOURNAL PAGES

To do: Week of_____ to _____

_____

_____

_____

_____

_____

Monday, _____ (On a scale of 1–10, how is my mood?)

_____

_____

_____

_____

_____

Tuesday, _____ (Are my medications working?)

_____

_____

_____

_____

_____

Wednesday, _____ (How is my spending going this week?)

_____

_____

_____

_____

_____

Thursday, _____ (Am I eating a bipolar-friendly diet?)

_____

_____

_____

_____

_____

Friday,_____ (How is my exercise this week?)

_____

_____

_____

_____

_____

Saturday,_____ (What can I do for fun today?)

_____

_____

_____

_____

_____

Sunday, _____ (How was my sleep this week?)

_____

_____

_____

_____

_____

Possible triggers this week:

_____

_____

_____

_____

_____

MOOD SWING MONITORING CHART

The chart on page 280 can help you to see patterns in your mood swings. Make copies so that you have a chart for each month. If you notice a big change in your moods as you keep this chart, write the trigger next to the change so that you can avoid the trigger in the future. If you're a woman, also note your menstrual cycle. If you have trouble with anger and aggression, look for a pattern. If you seem to get depressed at certain times of the day, note this in the chart. You can also write down when you start or stop a medication so that you can see the results. Put a dot on the graph to represent your mood each day. Dots on the line mean that you are feeling normal; dots below represent depression, while dots above indicate mania. Make sure that you note any of the other major bipolar disorder symptoms you are experiencing, such as psychosis or anxiety, as well. At the end of the month, you can then connect the dots for a graph of your moods. Opposite, is an example of a mood swing chart for ultrarapid cycling Bipolar II.

Month: *September* Year: *2005*

Mood Swing Monitoring Chart

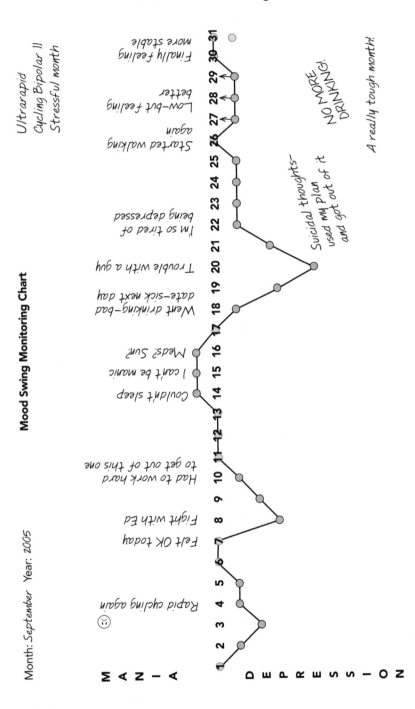

Ultrarapid Cycling Bipolar II Stressful month

Finally feeling more stable

Low—but feeling better

Started walking again

I'm so tired of being depressed

Trouble with a guy

Went drinking—bad date—sick next day

Meds? Sun?

I can't be manic

Couldn't sleep

Had to work hard to get out of this one

Fight with Ed

Felt OK today

Rapid cycling again

Suicidal thoughts— used my plan and got out of it

NO MORE DRINKING!

A really tough month!

M A N I A

D E P R E S S I O N

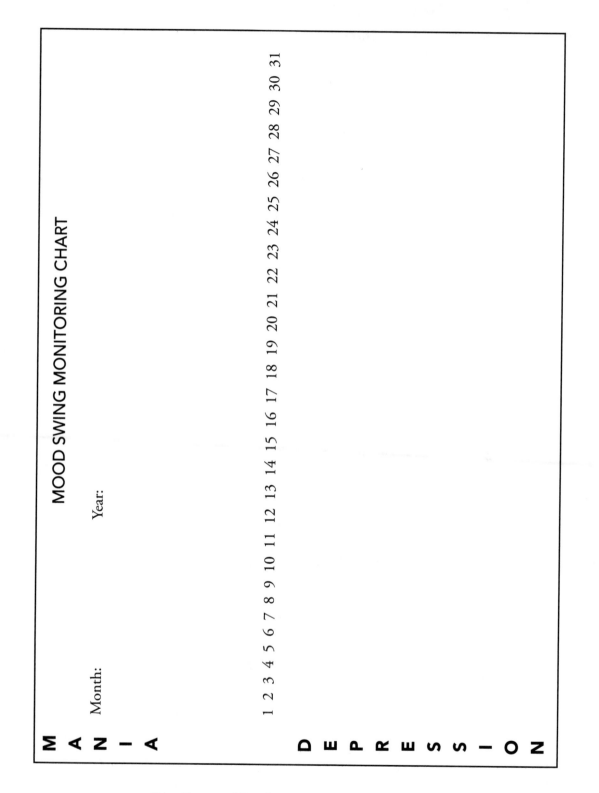

MOOD SWING MONITORING CHART

Month: Year:

M
A
N
I
A

1 2 3 4 5 6 7 8 9 10 11 12 13 14 15 16 17 18 19 20 21 22 23 24 25 26 27 28 29 30 31

D
E
P
R
E
S
S
I
O
N

Take Charge of Bipolar Disorder/Warner Wellness

ENDNOTES

Introduction. What Is Bipolar Disorder?

1. Akiskal, H. S. and Bourgeois, M. L., et al. (2000) Re-evaluating the prevalence of and diagnostic composition within the broad clinical spectrum of bipolar disorders. *J. Affective Disorders,* 59, Suppl: S5–530; Judd, L., Akiskal, H. S., Schettler, P. J., et al. (2002) The long-term natural history of the weekly symptomatic status of bipolar I disorder. *Arch Gen Psychiatry,* 59: 530–537.
2. American Psychiatric Association (2002) Practice Guidelines for the Treatment of Patients with Bipolar Disorder: Revised. Washington, D.C.: 18.
3. Ibid.

Chapter 1. Medications and Supplements

1. Bowden, C. L. and Singh, V. (2005) Long-term management of bipolar disorder. In: *Advances in the Treatment of Bipolar Disorder.* Edited by T. A. Ketter, American Psychiatric Publishing, Washington, D.C., p. 135.
2. Gitlin, M. (2002) Depression Myths and Contrary Realities. Continuing Education Series, UCLA.
3. Kessler, R. C., et al. (1994) Lifetime and 12-month prevalence of DSM III-R psychiatric disorders in the United States: Results from the National Co-morbidity Study. *Archives of General Psychiatry.* 51: 8–19.
4. Stoll, et al., *Archives of General Psychiatry.* 56 (1999): 407–412.
5. Nemets, et al., *American Journal of Psychiatry* 159 (2002): 477–479.
6. Pope, M. and Scott, J. (2003) Do clinicians understand why individuals stop taking lithium? *J. Affective Disorders,* 74, 287–291.

7. NIMH (2000) Bipolar Disorder Research: NIMH. http://www.nimh.nih.gov/publicat/NIMHbipolarresfact.pdf; Nurnberger, J. (in progress) Collaborative genomic study of bipolar disorder: NIMH grant number 1R01MH59545-01.

Chapter 2. Sleep, Diet, Exercise, and Light

1. Wurtman, J. (1986) *Managing Your Mind and Mood Through Food.* Rawson Associates, New York.
2. Dey, S. (1994) Physical exercise as a novel antidepressant agent: possible role of serotonin receptor subtypes. *Physiological Behavior* 55(2): 323–29; Norden, M. J. (1995) *Beyond Prozac.* Regan Books, New York
3. Malkoff-Schwartz, S., Frank, E., et al., (1998) Stressful life events and social rhythm disruption in the onset of manic depressive bipolar episodes: A preliminary investigation. *Archives of Gen. Psych.,* 55, 702–707.

Chapter 6. Choosing a Supportive Health Care Team

1. *The American Psychiatric Press Textbook of Psychiatry,* third edition.
2. "Bipolar Disorder," publication number 01-3679, National Institute of Mental Health, Bethesda, MD (2001).
3. Perry, A., Tamier, N., et al., (1999) Randomized controlled trial of efficacy of teaching patients with bipolar disorder to identify early symptoms of relapse and obtain treatment. *British Med. Journal,* 318, 149–153.
4. American Psychiatric Association (2002) Practice Guidelines for the Treatment of Patients with Bipolar Disorder: Revised. Washington D.C.
5. Ibid., 37.

INDEX

ABOUT THE AUTHORS

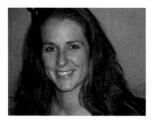

Julie A. Fast was diagnosed with ultrarapid cycling Bipolar II in 1995 after fifteen years of constantly wondering, *What's wrong with me? Why can't I stay in one job, maintain relationships, or live in one place?* Her partner of ten years was diagnosed with Bipolar I in 1994. She believes that this gives her books a very unique perspective. Her philosophy is that bipolar disorder is not the chaotic mess it seems, but is instead a very predictable and often very treatable illness once a person finds the right treatment plan. Her dream is that all people with bipolar disorder find a management system that works for them individually, so that they can have happy, healthy, and stable lives. Her main goal is to change the way the world sees and treats bipolar disorder: she believes that people with bipolar disorder have an illness, not psychological or personal problems. Julie manages the Web sites www.bipolarhappens.com and www.juliefast.com and is also the author, along with John Preston, of the bestselling *Loving Someone with Bipolar Disorder: Understanding and Helping Your Partner* (New Harbinger, 2004).

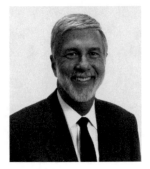

John Preston, PsyD, ABPP, is a professor of psychology with Alliant International University, Sacramento. He has also taught on the faculty of the UC Davis School of Medicine. Dr. Preston is the author of seventeen books, with topics including psychotherapy, depression, psychopharmacology, and neurobiology, and wrote the "Drugs in Psychiatry" chapter in *Encyclopedia Americana.* He has lectured in the United States, Europe, and Russia.